Jar

How to survive cancer

ANTI CANCER TREATMENTS

Prevention | Therapies | Aftercare

including
proton & carbon ion
radiotherapy

The original German edition was published in 2016 under the title
"Krebs innovativ geheilt – Vorsorgen | Heilen | Nachsorgen"

Image rights to author's photo: Dr Thomas Kästenbauer
Image rights to book cover: Mag. Janina Collin – special thanks to Georg
Translater: Martina Lammers
Graphics: Maria-Michaela V. Borejko

ISBN Print: 978-1-549731-63-1

E-Mail: krebs.innovativ.geheilt@gmail.com
www.krebsinnovativgeheilt.com

Layout, typesetting and production: Janina Collin – special thanks to Georg

For all mothers,
who tirelessly fight
for their children's health.

For all (marriage) partners
who make every day special
with their infinite love.

Contents

Prologue

My birth was uncomplicated, I was neither premature nor late and the first of three children. My mother keeps emphasising that I had kept strictly to her development schedule.

I was breastfed, had regular naps and feeds and was full of energy in my infancy and youth.

So far pretty much everyone in my family had lived to a ripe old age. My great-grandparents and my grandparents had averaged 90 without any great exertion. Cancer had never been an issue – until the diagnosis that would turn my life upside down.

None of us had anticipated my sickness, but apparently cancer can afflict anyone. Sinister storm clouds suddenly appeared on a radiantly blue sky.

But why did the sudden cancer verdict surprise me so much? The body has to fight millions of precursor cells on a daily basis. Does it therefore not nearly stand to reason that some people will sooner or later suffer from cancer? Statistics, too, prove me right. According to a WHO survey as early as 2012, 14.1 million people worldwide were already newly diagnosed with the disease. In western countries every third person in his or her lifetime will be afflicted by it. And tendencies are rising.

Usually a healthy, sound immune system handles the daily onslaught of stimulants quiet well and we don't pay much attention. We do not really consider and appreciate how extremely well our body performs on a daily basis, until we are suddenly, directly or indirectly, confronted with cancer.

In 2010 I was a newly diagnosed cancer patient who, compared to today, had little medical knowledge and initially felt powerlessly and helplessly abandoned to my fate and as close to every second cancer patient dies and the doctors gave me barely any hope of recovery, I realised that I had to mobilise all my strength and fight for my life myself. I had been raised not to give up when faced with difficulties. As the sayings go: Nothing ventured nothing gained and who dares wins.

And thus extensive research, numerous doctor appointments, stamina, obstinacy and certainly also a bit of luck led me to an innovative, medically recognised therapy. My degree course in biological psychology, already providing me with insights into the body's medical processes, as well as my mind-set of critically questioning any assertions no matter how renowned the source, also helped. I would now like to share the experience and knowledge gained during my elaborate research with those who have neither the strength nor the time to find their way through the jungle of various options.

By now I have presumably explored the subject of cancer, its treatments as well as pre- and post-operative care, more intensively than most physicians. For me the subject is not a profession – it is my life.

Janina Collin, September 2017

Why I wrote this book

When I was diagnosed with cancer my whole world initially collapsed around me. At the young age of 28 the doctors wanted to remove all nerve fibres from the right side of my face to combat salivary gland cancer. I would never again have been able to eat, speak and close one of my eyes properly. Optically disfigured, I would still not have been guaranteed a full recovery. Instead of agreeing to the surgical procedure I decided I would rather die. The decision was extremely difficult and at first plunged my family into an evidently severe crisis. But then it also released enormous amounts of energy, particularly in my mother and myself because basically all of us humans want the same: TO LIVE! Through much dedication, commitment and luck I found the type of therapy best suited to me and could therefore spare myself an operation with a clear conscience, not least towards my family. The search for the appropriate therapy raised numerous issues to which hardly anyone could or wanted to supply the answers.

In this book I will present meticulously gathered research in comprehensible terms. Amongst other subjects I will address the possibilities of conventional treatments such as chemotherapy, surgery, immunotherapy and various radiotherapies. I also aim to convey in an easily understandable way to those seeking help, how dietary supplements' curative powers have convinced me when accompanying orthodox treatments but particularly during aftercare. Only when we realise how nutritional supplements beneficially affect our body are we motivated enough to take them. While selecting them, I trusted my research, personal evaluation and gut feeling. Today, seven years after my radiation therapy, I finally feel well again and I can optimistically look towards the future.

This book has been written for all those who endeavour to become healthy or stay healthy. I wish to ease the path for those afflicted and their relatives and to encourage them to evaluate their own options to overcome the disease.

Tracing the symptoms

It was the spring of 2010 when I first felt sure that something wasn't quite right. For close to the past two years twitching and slight asymmetries had developed in my face which I had initially attributed to the stress associated with a previous chapter in my life and the unpleasant confines of a past relationship. Meanwhile I had ended the affair, dealt with a budding herpes simplex virus and periodic bouts of fever. I had also had some excellent herbal teas prepared for me by a practitioner of Chinese medicine. Her acupuncture needles played their part as well, but nothing helped in the long term. Apart from temporary improvements my facial problems had steadily increased. No matter how hard I tried, I could not explain the cause of my medical complaints. I had entered into a new relationship I considered a great gift. A wonderful man by my side now, I was full of vitality, everything fitted and we started planning our future together. So why did those facial tics and asymmetries still persist?

In May I finally braced myself and visited a renowned facial paralysis specialist. I don't particularly like going to the doctor and therefore asked my mother to accompany me. This gave me support and, what's more, the opportunity to jointly deliberate and discuss the doctor's visit afterwards. In my view the subsequent examinations didn't seem focused. The doctor tapped some facial areas, checked my reflexes and my sense of balance. I instantly knew that he wouldn't find anything conspicuous. After all, I would surly have noticed if anything was wrong with my sensations and responses two years on. These examinations therefore proved useless. I really needed to discover the reasons for my facial nerve paralysis and the increasingly severe vellication (nervous spasms). So the doctor sent me for further check-ups: magnetic resonance imaging (MRI) of the brain, a blood test and a nerve conduction velocity (NCV) test. The blood tests results came back first and were normal. I hadn't expected anything else as I felt quite healthy overall. The MRI images also didn't show anything noticeable. Looking back I now understand why the MRI hadn't revealed the tumour as it had merely examined the brain but not the spot behind the ear which hurt. This left the NCV.

Instinctively as well as objectively assessing the situation, I thought this test would expose the first hidden deficiencies to everyone and consequently be a step in the right direction. My symptoms were of a neuronal nature and now, I believed, we were beginning to find the causes. I felt a hard to describe inner tension. On the one hand I somehow looked forward to finally proving there actually was something wrong and I wasn't just being vain – something I had also been accused of as my facial paralysis hadn't been particularly pronounced at that stage. On the other I was scared of the diagnosis as it would soon be a certainty that something had gotten out of hand. For the test, surface patch electrodes are placed on the skin. The nerves are stimulated with electrical impulses. If they are healthy, they typically react quickly with facial distortions and muscle contractions. These can be measured, analysed and compared to the norm. Should a particular part of the face not react, however, this indicates an anomaly. I found the procedure uncomfortable and painful, but bravely endured it, consoling myself with the all-important moment of truth. The test showed that my facial nerves had lost approximately 70 percent of their function. Naturally I asked the doctor who had performed the procedure about his opinion. He stated that he could merely confirm the reduced nerve function, but possible causes would have to be discussed with my referring physician. Going back to my alleged facial nerve paralysis specialist I now hoped the findings would be meticulously analysed. My mother and I felt relieved when we entered the practice and found no other patients in the waiting room. Apparently a lot of time had been reserved for my case. And so I anticipated an extensive consultation in which the secret of my physical condition would finally be revealed. Shortly before being called into the surgery, however, the next patient arrived and I wondered how long she'd have to wait. I got my answer sooner than expected. To our great amazement the doctor curtly informed me that everything was within the normal range. A facial nerve paralysis occasionally occurred for no apparent reason. Although I was still young at 28, he continued, I would have to live with the condition. That that was just the way it was.

Staring at my equally surprised mother I tried to digest his outrageous statement. With difficulty I controlled my burgeoning indignation. Then, having calmed down, yet still close to tears, I reminded the man of the symptomatic and increasingly unpleasant facial problems. In the process I once more addressed the fact that I'd had an inexplicable pain behind my ear for years, which now, in combination with the facial paralysis, caused me grave concern. But those arguments didn't move him at all. In his opinion this was entirely unrelated to the paralysis. Since the pain had presented before the paralysis, a connection could be completely ruled out, anyway. So I shouldn't get into such a state about the matter and accept things as they were. Besides, he told us in no uncertain terms, it was time for us to please leave now as the next patient was waiting. Totally unprepared for the turn the conversation had taken, I speechlessly leaned back in my chair. My mother now spoke up and made it clear that I was certainly not getting worked up over nothing. The problem had, after all, started two years ago and had become more and more severe. For that reason, she explained, before something even worse might happen, I had visited his surgery for clarification of the symptoms. She got right to the heart of the matter. But the doctor was not prepared to prolong the discussion. His final, laconic comment – somewhat irritated, but succinct – would end the consultation: "Men don't just look for a symmetrical face! I strongly advise you to leave it at that!"

I was shocked. I wasn't here because I was worried about landing a boyfriend but because I sensed deep down that there was something wrong with my health. Even on the way out of the consultation room the first tears started rolling down my cheeks. What a setback. What a disappointment!

The rest was pure formality: payment in full, no invoice and I just stood there, numb. We made it as far as the car when I was seized by a crying fit. My mother tried to console me. In my panic I sobbed, asking her what we should do next. Now I also had to convince my mother that the doctor was wrong and we had to keep looking for solutions. My mother was torn between believing that everything was alright and my deep conviction that everything was absolutely not alright.

My odyssey begins

Back home I sat down in front of the computer, browsed through medical directories and found an otolaryngologist (an ear, nose and throat specialist) whose CV and photo very much appealed to me and who seemed competent. I made an appointment for that same week and then I immersed myself in my research of facial nerve paralysis. I started to suspect the pressure pain behind my ear could be caused by a tumour. Soon I discovered a well-structured chart with possible causes and symptoms. One column surprisingly described all my symptoms including pressure pain. Sadly my suspicion of a tumour therefore intensified.

I was very happy with the doctor I had chosen. She was extremely friendly, took her time, listened patiently, explored my problem and quickly realised where I should proceed from here. A radiologist, who had been recommended by several people, conducted a further MRI of my head and neck area as well as an ultrasound diagnosis of the neck and ear – and finally found something! On the images he discovered something in the region of my parotid gland that shouldn't have been there. He, as well as my otolaryngologist, therefore advised a histological analysis. The otolaryngologist patiently explained how she would perform the biopsy – a more than four inch long incision past the ear down to the neck. The idea was so unpleasant to me, we agreed on a final observation period of about three months. We both took the risk involved in the delay as the suspected parotid tumour had apparently nestled cosily in my body for quite some time and had basically not led to a rapid deterioration. She did, however, advise me that urgent treatment would be required if I experienced any pain.

Within the agreed observation period, just as I began to hope that the growth wasn't malignant, I started feeling pains I had never felt before. They started from the ear and stretched over the entire right side of the neck.

This was new.

Initially my mother suspected dental problems probably affecting the area and was therefore not unduly worried. To me it felt like a hard, extremely tense muscle in my neck. At times the pain got so intense I didn't even know how to hold my head. Only when lying down slightly massaging the muscle was it somewhat more bearable. I was worried because the otolaryngologist had emphatically warned me: "Pain is an alarm signal!" But as the pain stopped again roughly a week later, I calmed down and postponed a further visit to the doctor. In any case, I was determined to go to the scheduled follow-up appointment.

The first concrete suspicion is voiced

Over the coming weeks my uncertainty increased. At this stage I could hardly wait for the follow-up appointment, I really needed clarity. Right after the examination the radiologist viewed my MRI images with me and very succinctly stated his suspicion. He talked of an *adenoid cystic carcinoma (ACC)* in the parotid gland. A rare, malignant tumour, especially present in the head and neck area, frequently emanating from the salivary glands to then spread through the surrounding tissue along the nerves. He pointed out that the only "redeeming grace" of this type of malignant cancer was that it grew relatively slowly and we therefore still had some time for in-depth research about possible treatment options before deciding how to proceed.

After all those weeks of worry and anxiety the radiologists suspected diagnosis still hit me hard. I felt as if somebody had pulled the rug out from under my feet; dizzy, nauseous and panicky. This was the moment everything was turned upside down.

In those days my life was rewritten. Much of what had previously been important vanished from my mind. Foundations collapsed. Standards changed.

The sky seemed more radiant than ever before and the birds' song simply beautiful. The colours of the sunsets were so magnificent, the atmosphere so romantic, I just couldn't get enough. Going to bed was a necessary evil, but the dawn with its tranquillity and the fresh, clean air quickly made up for the long, dark nights. Suddenly I experienced nature far more intensively and asked myself how many more of these magic moments I would be privileged to witness.

On the day of the suspected diagnosis my partner Georg had already arranged a get-together with his pals in the evening. He sat down beside me, hugged me and said: "I'll cancel tonight's meeting with the boys!" It was very tempting to continue being hugged and comforted by him. In the afternoon we cuddled on the sofa. Tears ran down our cheeks while we discussed a lot of issues. But then I realised what I wanted Georg to do. "Please see your friends. Have a good time together. I can cry on my own and I think it's better if you go out. When you come back you can make me laugh and distract me with some funny stories about your night out. That way life's still worth living." So I asked him to have some fun and return with a smile. It can't have been easy for him to leave me on my own on that fateful day. But I simply needed him to do that so I wouldn't drown in my sorrow and then give in to despair. Crying together, I realised, is important for a while but would not further my recovery.

To this day I can feel Georg's love and how precious I am to him. The time I get to spend with him is an invaluable gift. So many couples separate after or during cancer treatment for the most varied reasons. These relationships don't prove equal to the challenge. I know of a woman who lost an eye during surgery. Her partner just couldn't cope and ended the relationship. Being left at a time when one most needs support is tragic. Frequently, however, the sick person initiates the separation because he or she wants to be in charge of his or her own life and enjoy it without having to consider the other half. And then there are those who wallow in self-pity and complain about having to live with a critically ill partner and regard themselves as victims.

But Georg was there for me right from the start without even a moment's hesitation. He not only deliberated the most unorthodox treatments with my mother and me, he also respected and support all my decisions.

For this reason I hold Georg in highest regard and particularly love for him.

The search for the right therapy starts

I kept up my internet research, this time with the keyword of the probable diagnosis: *adenoid cystic carcinoma (ACC)*, and tried coming to terms with it. At first I didn't find much. Merely two other affected people who had chatted on an online forum. Both of them close to death at this stage. They talked about the countless therapies they

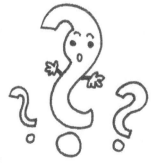

had tried in their desperation, alas without success. The insights gained by my research initially made me feel pretty despondent and powerless. Secretly I thought let it be anything but this! As soon as I had voiced the thought, I already regretted doing so. Even in childhood I had learned that I often got the things I wanted the least. I didn't like freckles, but once I said it, they already adorned my face. Physical asymmetries – no, thanks! The moment I thought about it, the first asymmetries in my face became apparent. Yes, I am vain, I honestly admit it. And I set myself high standards. And now? People wrote in an online forum that half the side of their face had been surgically removed and their cancer still hadn't been beaten. The possibility that I was suffering from the same medical condition and shared the same fate was so shocking that I abandoned my internet research for a period of time. My mother and I now started visiting various physicians to inform ourselves about the further procedure in case the suspected diagnosis turned out to be true. Back then we hadn't the slightest idea how difficult it would be to find the appropriate therapy. Many cancer patients blindly trust the recommendations of the first doctor they consult during the diagnostic stage. Most doctors encourage the patient with statements like: "You'll be alright. Cancer is not a death sentence." One can only hope those doctors are thoroughly familiar with the various treatments and suggest the most appropriate one.

The journey to find the most suitable therapy would turn out to be a difficult, rocky and prolonged one.

My mother was frequently at the computer for nights on end to jubilantly share her insights into the prospective "right" treatment. For a long time I simply commented with: "no" and "that's out of the question."

None of her suggestions appealed to my gut feelings and made proper sense to me! I wanted to live, but, above all, in a way that was *worth living.*

Today, based on my own experience, I realise the importance of selecting the right treatment from the outset. It's like competing in the Dakar Rally. You have to make the proper choices right from the start, in particular selecting the best racing car. The first stage is the most important. Those who don't manage it lose a lot of time. Then it gets difficult! I won the first lap by choosing the right vehicle for the terrain: the right therapy. I found it with my mother's help and a lot of luck.

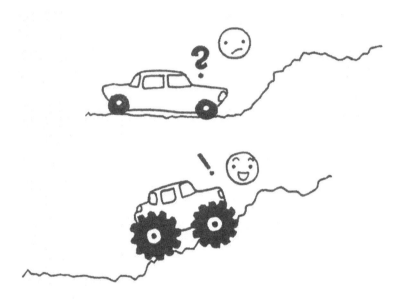

Now I know that a holistic treatment plan needs to be developed for the best feasible results. This is also aided by the patients extensively informing themselves about their options, which is only possible to learn from other people's experiences. An acutely affected patient often doesn't have the time and especially not the physical strength to "just try" chemotherapy, for instance, and change to another type of treatment if it doesn't work.

The choice requires extensive knowledge. And the sooner the right therapy is started, the higher the chances of returning back to health.

Cancer does not have to be a death sentence – if it is diagnosed in time and properly treated. With the appropriate concept most types of cancer afford a good chance of survival. The first five years after contracting the disease are the most critical. If this hurdle has been overcome the odds are in favour of more cancer-free years provided the patient adopts the right lifestyle.

Exploring conventional medical options

During my journey to find the best suitable therapy I explored the various conventional medical options. Here I will try to explain their effects and potential applications in understandable terms:

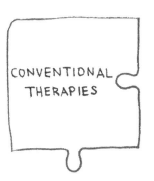

- Chemotherapy
- Cancer immunotherapy
- Surgery
- Radiotherapy

Chemotherapy – how it works

Try picturing a pond with water lilies. They multiply exponentially like tumour cells. One cell becomes 2, 2 cells become 4, 4 become 8, then 16, 32, 64 and so on.

Just like a pond only half covered with water lilies one

day can be completely covered with them the next, a tumour grows with increasing size and more and more rapidly. Chemotherapy utilises this reproduction strategy. The goal of chemotherapy is to arrest the tu-  mour's growth process by disrupting the tumour cells' metabolism or destroying the malignant cancer cells about to divide by damaging their genes. This is meant to induce the cancer cells to commit suicide, referred to as apoptosis (programmed cell death), which leads to the tumour shrinking and, at best, disappearing.

To that end *cytostatic drugs* (substances having a toxic effect on cells) are administered by intravenous infusion or in tablet form. Roughly thirty different cytostatic agents are currently available. However, the chemical substances can generally not be administered to the tumour alone. They therefore don't just destroy the dividing malignant cells but also dividing benign cells – with all the associated short- as well as long-term side effects.

The short term ones affect the blood cells, the mucous membrane, the skin and the hair roots. This can result in anaemia, susceptibility to infections and hair loss. The long term side effects, depending on the cytostatic drugs administered and their dosage, include long-term damages to nearly all the organs such as the kidneys, heart and liver, the nervous system and the bones. As beneficial as chemotherapy may be for some types of cancer, some tumours sadly can't be treated with it. Therefore a chemosensitivity test should, if possible, be conducted beforehand. Essentially chemotherapy is more effective the faster the cancer cells divide.

Many cytostatic drugs used in chemotherapy reduce the production of white and red blood cells in the bone marrow. A low white blood cell count, however, renders the human body susceptible to viral, bacterial or fungal infections which can be life- threatening to the weakened immune system. Doctors can counteract this negative development with drugs which stimulate the production of white blood cells again. These drugs are mostly injected under the skin or administered intravenously. Unfortunately they also frequently cause side effects so that the pros and cons will have to be carefully evaluated.

It is imperative to bear in mind that cytostatic agents not only destroy cancer cells but also reproductive cells, i.e. ova and sperm cells, depending on the type and dosage.

Those who want to have children in the future should therefore discuss the issue with a medical professional as there are ways of preventing potential infertility.

In my case of *adenoid cystic carcinoma (ACC)* the tumour cells were dividing quite slowly. The benefits (the eradication of relatively few cancer cells) wouldn't have outweighed the damage inflicted by chemotherapy (such as a weakened immune system). I therefore ruled it out as a treatment option. Looking back, and after having met some ACC sufferers who had chemotherapy without any positive effects whatsoever, I'm very happy with my decision.

For some kinds of cancer, particularly *chronic myeloid leukaemia*, chemotherapy is still the method of choice. For some years now there's been a drug on the market which heals chronic myeloid leukaemia. It causes the cancer cells to die after a few weeks if taken orally on a daily basis. The drug invades the receptors through which the cancer cells recharge their energy and thus robs the cancer of its growth advantage over healthy cells.

For other types of leukaemia, such as *acute lymphoblastic leukemia*, where sufferers were practically considered to be hopeless cases after a relapse, hope now exists through immunotherapy.

Immunotherapy – a wake-up call for the immune system

Cancer immunotherapy comprises various immunotherapy methods to fight cancer. Instead of directly attacking the cancer cells the immune system is strengthened. We differentiate between active and passive immunotherapy. During *active immunotherapy* the patient is prescribed substances aimed at causing an immune response which triggers the death of the tumour cells. During *passive immunotherapy* the patient is given antibodies or antibody particles.

These antibodies are artificially produced and can help in treating cancer through the immune system attacking the tumour cells while the healthy cells are spared. Some antibodies attach themselves to the cancer cells' surfaces in the process and send signals to the immune system to destroy them. Other antibodies appear to provoke some kind of suicide programme in the usually indestructible tumour cells. Others again obstruct receptors that serve the cancer cells to latch on. For some years now there's also been the approach of disrupting signalling pathways in cancer cells. This inhibits growth signals conducted from the cell surface to the cell nucleus. Antibody therapies can curb tumour growth. Admittedly though it doesn't yet seem possible to eliminate all the tumour cells. For that reason antibody therapy is frequently combined with chemotherapy.

Good results are currently being achieved in some forms of lymphoma, bowel cancer, bladder cancer, renal cancer, triple negative breast cancer, malignant melanoma, stomach cancer or lung cancer in some cases.

In 2017 Dr Behnam Badie, City of Hope Comprehensive Cancer Center in Duarte, CA, was the first doctor who was able to successfully treat brain tumours like glioblastoma using immunotherapy. He and his team will make further studies.

With *adoptive immunotherapy*, already successfully applied in acute lymphoblastic leukaemia, defence cells are extracted from the patient and manipulated in the lab in a way that they more readily recognise and fight cancer cells. After the modified cells have multiplied in a bioreactor for ten days, they are returned to the patient through an infusion. They now attack a protein on the degenerated white blood cells' surface. The first acute lymphoblastic leukaemia patients treated with this method have already been cancer-free for four years.

The approach that the body's own defence cells are able to fight tumours is at present being intensively researched. For their fight against cancer the T-cells – white blood cells for immune defence – are equipped with a genetically engineered "sensor" (CAR receptor) so they recognise a certain molecule in the cancer cells. The right sensor has to be found for the particular cancer type.

Further research and authorisation procedures are required for these concepts to be applied in the treatment of several cancer types.

Cancer usually develops when, for various reasons, the immune system has become weakened or unable to recognise the cancer cells. I therefore feel this is a promising approach towards treating cancer through "artificially" influencing the immune system. Having said this, immunotherapy, the new ray of hope, also has side effects as it induces an autoimmune reaction with varied symptoms in the body.

> → **My Advice:** Anyone diagnosed with cancer, particularly with a rare or hard to treat type, should send their own reports and MRI images to several renowned clinics, if possible worldwide, to enquire about treatment options and prognoses.

Immuno- and antibody therapy was not possible to treat my kind of tumour. So I had to research the third orthodox medical option: surgery.

Surgery – the radical solution

During surgery the tumour is removed together with some of the surrounding healthy tissue to minimise the risk of leaving abnormal tissue behind. At best the tumour is well isolated from the healthy tissue and therefore easily removable. This is practically always the case with benign tumours as they are encapsulated from the adjacent tissue. Malignant tumours, however, frequently grow in an infiltrating manner. This means they don't confine themselves to a defined area but "stretch their limbs" to spread to wherever they feel "comfortable". My type of tumour for instance, the *adenoid cystic carcinoma (ACC)*, likes being close to glands and nerves. But it doesn't just grow alongside them, it also infiltrates them and investigates further areas, even "jumps" at times. For this reason the surgery is radical and extensive. Should the tumour be close to vital organs a complete surgical removal creates an immense challenge and may even be impossible. And, what's worse, a visual distinction between cancerous and healthy tissue is frequently extremely difficult.

Therefore, "to be on the safe side", radiotherapy is performed in addition to the operation. But radiation treatment should be considered very carefully, especially if the tumour was completely removed. Should another tumour appear in the treated area at a later stage, repeated radiation may have to be denied if the highest possible dosage will be exceeded.

Occasionally it is also attempted to shrink a tumour through radio- or chemotherapy so it can be operated on. The decreased amount of cancer cells reduces the probability of the tumour's relapse (recurrence after its radical removal or complete remission) and the formation of metastases (the tumour invading other parts of the body).

Preoperative radiation can also damage the cancer cells to the extent that tumours, which are highly manipulated during surgery, can no longer shed any metastasising cells.

Hormone treatment – an additional option

Additional hormone treatment is often recommended after cancer surgery.

In the case of cancer, hormone treatment should really be called "anti-hormonal treatment" as it is intended to suppress the development of endogenous hormones which allow certain cancer types to grow.

Therefore hormone treatment is employed for highly sensitive tumours such as prostate cancer or sometimes breast and uterus cancer. These tumour cells have special binding sites, so-called hormone receptors. Their growth is inadvertently encouraged by certain endogenous hormones and has to be prohibited. There are various options:

- surgical removal of hormone production areas such as the ovaries or testicles,
- medical suppression of the endogenous hormone production or
- blocking hormone action with a hormone receptor modulator. This attaches to the tumour cells and blocks them without developing hormone action itself.

31

One has to consider that hormone therapies are aimed at eliminating sex hormones which entails certain consequences. Generally cancer can't be cured by hormone treatment alone. It merely retards the growth. Therefore it can only be recommended as an additional measure to increase the chances of recovery.

However, over time hormone-sensitive tumours can develop a resistance to hormone treatment and thus render it useless. The pros and cons must therefore be carefully examined. For me it was not an option as my type of cancer, adenoid cystic carcinoma (ACC), is most likely not hormone dependent.

Gathering specific information regarding surgery

On the internet I found a resident doctor at Cologne University Hospital who was supposed to specialise in adenoid cystic carcinoma surgery. So I decided to fly to Cologne to quiz him about his approach.

During the consultation he explained his proposed surgical procedure. He would open up the affected neck area to gain an overview. If I really had a malignant tumour, which would be determined during surgery by a pathological examination, he would radically remove the entire tumour including its offshoots. This would also entail the surgical resection of the facial nerve with all its branches. This extensive surgical intervention would have meant that the entire right side of my face would no longer function. I would be unable to properly laugh, eat, speak, drink and close my right eye. At my young age I would not only be optically disfigured but also heavily impaired in my daily life. According to the specialist nerve reconstruction surgery could be performed but there was naturally no guarantee that the new nerve would take root and assume sensory or motoric functions. My own research showed that nerve reconstruction surgery would probably only achieve a so-called hibernation mode. The best case scenario for me would have been that my face was reasonably symmetrical when passive. But that was about as much as I could have hoped for. The idea was downright depressing, particularly as it would not have guaranteed being cured despite complex surgery. Surgical intervention was unimaginable to me on an emotional level. Even back then I suffered from parts of my facial expressions no longer functioning and the existence of this merely symmetrical resting state. Other functions of the right side of my face were already restricted and made it inconceivable to surgically remove the entire facial nerve with all its precious remaining functions!

After leaving the doctor's surgery my mother and I still decided to enjoy an afternoon in Cologne despite the difficult situation we were facing. We strolled through the city until we eventually ended up in Cologne's famous cathedral where we spotted a wish box in a side aisle. We wrote our wish on a slip of paper – to discover the right treatment – and put it into the box. Despite the depressing consultation with the specialist and for no objective reason I felt slightly more optimistic that an acceptable solution would be found.

To round off the day we treated ourselves with refreshments at a café. For quite a while now I had denied myself carbohydrates and sugar. But that day I enjoyed a cup of hot chocolate. Some of my vitality returned, feeling reinvigorated, and a little high on sugar, we strolled back to the hotel.

We agreed that surgery would have to be avoided at all costs. The predicted downsides made the best possible end result look so terribly bad that this option could only be considered as an emergency solution. We now had to search for an alternative treatment option which would successfully restore my health without surgical intervention.

Histology (tissue analysis) provides clarity

Up to this point in time we didn't have a histological diagnosis. I had started all my previous research based on the MRI and ultrasound findings, my discernable facial symptoms and my gut instincts. The physician I had visited in Cologne therefore urged me to have a tissue sample analysis to provide absolute clarity. He told me that instead of a four inch incision in the ear-neck region, diagnostically conclusive tissue material could be obtained through a needle biopsy. Back at home I went to a clinic in Vienna to make an appointment with a competent ENT physician to conduct such a biopsy.

I had already informed myself about the procedure. A thin, hollow, needle is inserted into the area to be analysed (fine needle aspiration) to extract continuous cell ranges. The samples are placed on a microscope slide for pathological examination. However, if not enough continuous cells have been removed or a small sample only contains inconspicuous cells, this could lead to a misdiagnosis.

My fine needle aspiration appointment was in November 2010. On arrival at the Vienna clinic I was directly referred to a radiologist. To my astonishment the radiologist was scheduled to perform the biopsy and not the ENT specialist of my choice. At my request, however, the ENT specialist was summoned to assist with the procedure. The radiologist used needles of various sizes and sucked three different samples from the suspect area near the parotid gland aided by ultrasound imaging. The punctures, particularly when he used the last and thickest needle, were extremely painful and I endured them with great difficulty. Only the prospect of clarity and the chance of avoiding major surgery made me persevere and increased my pain threshold.

I now focused on the results and could hardly wait for the pathologist's assessment. But the disappointing verdict was that no contiguous tissue could be obtained from the samples and a diagnosis was therefore impossible.

Because I wanted to leave no stone unturned and my research had discovered that certain cancer types can also be detected through a pregnancy test, I took one. The result was negative. The test didn't reveal a pregnancy and therefore also no tumour. Once more I briefly felt hopeful that I was healthy after all – but the signs clearly contradicted this.

By now I know why in some cases cancer can quite easily be verified by a pregnancy test. Some types of cancer generate sufficient *pre-embryonic trophoblasts* (cell layers normally responsible for the later-stage embryo's nutrition). They, in turn, produce the pregnancy hormone (Beta-)hCG (human chorionic gonadotropin) which can be detected by a Beta-hCG pregnancy test. These types of tumours include those stemming from the placenta or germ cells of the ovaries or testicles.

As my kind of cancer, the adenoid cystic carcinoma (ACC) doesn't generate any or not sufficient pre-embryonic trophoblasts it, like many other cancer types, can not be detected by a pregnancy test.

So I had no choice but to undergo another needle biopsy two weeks later, this time in the hospital's outpatient clinic. Equipped with only two needles my ENT specialist extracted further samples from the throat area in question and was convinced that he'd now obtained contiguous tissue. He was in fact successful and some days later I received the histological confirmation of malignant cell proliferation in the area of my parotid gland.

I now had to accept the sad reality that I suffered from a malignant tumour. Unfortunately the specific type of cancer could not be determined from the extracted tissue samples as not enough contiguous tissue was present. This should soon make me face further challenges.

The search for the right therapy continues...

Radical surgery, i.e. the removal of the parotid gland as well as the entire facial nerve was utterly out of the question. So my mother helped me with the research into alternative ways of tumour management.

Radiotherapy under the spotlight

After I had ruled out the conventional treatments chemotherapy, immunotherapy and surgery, I decided to take a more in-depth look at radiotherapy.

Could this be the treatment that would cure me?

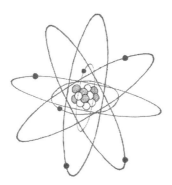

Cancer is the second most common cause of death in Europe. Roughly half of those diagnosed are "healed" through orthodox methods such as surgery, chemotherapy or ionising radiation with electrons or photons. A patient is deemed to be healed if the treatment results in five years of being tumour-free.

The other half of cancer cases cannot (as yet) be cured, either because the metastases proliferate or the tumour cannot be entirely destroyed at its source although no metastases are as yet present. This is the case, for instance, when the tumour is sited very close to vital organs, resistant to chemotherapeutic substances or radiation types established in tumour treatment.

I now had to find a radiotherapy that could destroy my barely treatable tumour: the most efficient and effective radiotherapy in existence which also perfectly preserved the surrounding tissue.

With those stipulations in mind I started informing myself about the various types of radiotherapy.

Radiation is either applied through external beam radiotherapy (also called *teletherapy*) or internally through *brachytherapy*.

X-rays, gamma rays and photon rays

Worldwide external radiation treatment is predominantly applied with high frequency gamma rays or x-rays. This is also called photon radiation. Photon radiation consists of electromagnetic waves such as radio waves, microwaves or light.

Nowadays electromagnetic radiations are mainly used in radiotherapy, however they are not always suitable for killing cancerous growths. As photon rays basically can't be accurately aimed, the tissue on each side and behind the tumour is exposed to high radiation levels during the attempt to apply a sufficiently high dose of radiation to the tumour.

Yet occasionally the radiation of the tumour's environment can actually be beneficial when cancer cells have already spread around the tumour.

To minimise the damage to the surrounding tissue as much as possible, the tumour is generally irradiated from different directions to apply as high a dose as possible to the malignant tissue, with minimal damage to the surrounding healthy tissue. This is referred to as *intensity modulated radiation therapy (IMRT)*. It was developed from *3D conformal radiation technology*, as IMRT can adjust the dose inside the target area as well as the shape of the irradiated area and the various irradiation angles.

Because the tumour's position between irradiation units can change (distinctly at times), for example through breathing or intestinal activity, state-of-the-art imaging techniques have been employed for some years now to facilitate immediate correction if a deviation from the original location occurs. Since radiation equipment has been supplemented by imaging techniques it is possible to view the patient's insides directly before the treatment, thus increasing its accuracy. This is called *image guided radiation therapy (IGRT)*.

A further development from IMRT is the *volumetric modulated arc therapy (VMAT)*. Here the radiation equipment rotates continuously around the patient during the treatment. This has further improved dose adjustment to the tumour and significantly reduced the irradiation times per unit as compared to IMRT. IGRT technology in correctly placing the patient and the target area also plays its role. Highly accurate, fractionated radiooncological treatment methods are usually divided into three to six irradiation units with individual doses of 8 to 20 Gray (symbol: Gy = radiation dose unit in radiotherapy). This is called *stereotactic radiotherapy (SRT)*. If the irradiation is a single high dose treatment it is referred to as *radiosurgery (SRS)* which employs advanced linear accelerators.

Stereotactic radiotherapy was originally developed for

treating small tumours in the head region. It was limited to those as coordinate points had to be screwed into the skull for accurate positioning and because tumours in the head region presented little risk of dislocation. Image guided radiation therapy has by now also paved the way for treatment of tumours in the trunk of the body.

Radiotherapy with photons is suitable for treating radiation-sensitive tumours and is available in many clinics. Equipment which can provide this high energy radiation is widespread all over the world and produced by various manufacturers. These linear accelerators are known under the registered trademarks Novalis, TX®, XKnife®, Axesse® and CyberKnife.

CyberKnife

CyberKnife is a robotic image guided radiation system whereby physicians can very accurately irradiate tumours with the aid of photon rays. The photons damage the cells' DNA so that they are ideally no longer able to divide. Tumours irradiated with CyberKnife can't be too large and have to be clearly segregated from the remaining tissue. With CyberKnife the entire dose is usually administered in a single treatment. If clinically required, however, the dose is also administered in two to five sessions. Each treatment takes between 60 and 90 minutes. Typical there are up to 1200 different radiation angles. Potential patients' movements are recognised by the robot-assisted system which reacts appropriately to correct them in order to keep irradiating the tumour with high precision.

By being irradiated from so many directions the surrounding healthy tissue is "spared" and the tumour destroyed where all the rays meet. Over the course of the following months the body then ideally breaks down the damaged, destroyed tumour. However, through the administered high dose of radiation over few treatments the probability of side effects increases. Especially in the brain, damages can have unpleasant consequences. CyberKnife can treat benign as well as malignant tumours. These include acoustic neuroma, meningioma, lung and liver cancer as well as metastases in the brain, the spine, the lungs and the liver.

Gamma Knife

I would also like to mention Gamma Knife which uses cobalt sources to generate gamma rays. Gamma Knife consists of a hemispheric helmet equipped with roughly 200 individual cobalt-60 radiation sources. It's design renders it mainly suitable for treating brain lesions. Tumours can be irradiated at each individual source. It takes between half an hour to two hours for the entire tumour to be irradiated in one treatment. Gamma Knife is a radiotherapy device developed by a Swedish company and primarily employed in the case of small brain tumours, brain metastases, meningioma and acoustic neuroma.

As adenoid cystic carcinoma is extremely resilient to gamma or photon rays respectively and therefore requires an extremely high absorbed dose to eliminate the tumour cells (tumour stem cells), the side effects usually increase immensely with a single high dose. I therefore ruled out CyberKnife and Gamma Knife as well as all the other forms of radiation involving photons described in this chapter. As a patient one absolutely has a say when choosing the therapy. It therefore stands to reason to educate oneself as much as possible. I now aimed to find a high-dose radiotherapy which accurately irradiated but was spread over many individual sessions. The lower the single dose per irradiation unit and the more accurate the irradiation, the less side effects could be expected.

At this stage I would like to point out that tissue which has already been irradiated may possibly not be irradiated again in case of renewed tumour growth if the total therapeutic dose would be exceeded.

The findings of a clinical study conducted by the Institute of Heavy Ion Research at Darmstadt in collaboration with the University of Heidelberg confirmed my view that photon radiation in patients with adenoid cystic carcinoma (ACC) was not the way to proceed. The local tumour control rate (i.e. the probability of a tumour's non-growth) is merely 24.6 percent four years later. This means that after exclusive photon irradiation (total dose 66 Gy) the tumour will return with a high probability of 75.4 percent.

Based on the by me rather accidentally researched high *recurrence rate* (the frequency in which a tumour presents again after its radical removal), I decided against photon irradiation despite experts' recommendations.

Knowing or not knowing can decide between life and death!

Only later did I discover in medical journals that radiotherapy utilising photons exclusively would no longer be ethically acceptable in the case of adenoid cystic carcinoma. The decision was based on the tumour's low radiation sensitivity and its recognised high likelihood of recurrence. Additionally, I would no longer be treatable in case of a recurrence as the maximum tolerable dose of radiation would already have been administered to the tissue. Surgery to the irradiated area would also have been extremely difficult because of the tissue's poor healing tendency. [Wannemacher, Debus & Wenz (2006): p. 169: Maligne Speicheldrüsentumoren *(Malignant Salivary Gland Tumours)*]

And yet several clinics offered me this treatment. They either had no other type of radiotherapy available or those who did have a therapy suitable for my tumour were temporarily booked out.

An entirely different local tumour control rate emerges for my type of illness if at least part of the radiation dose is administered with carbon ions instead of photons. With this treatment the local tumour control rate is 77.5 percent after four years (compared to the 24.6 percent of exclusive photon irradiation described above). This means that the probability of the tumour returning is significantly lower at 22.5 percent when a combination of photons (54 Gy) and carbon ions (18 Gy) is applied.

Brachytherapy (short distance therapy)

Brachytherapy (Greek "brachys" = brief or short) is a type of radiotherapy where the radiation source, a radioactive compound, is placed a short distance from or within the tumour. Thus the tumour can be treated with high-dose local irradiation with little damage to healthy tissue. This is done with the aid of seed-like or pellet-like gamma emitters. Preferably used are iridium emitters (gamma emitters) but beta emitters such as yttrium and iodine isotopes are also deployed.

In terms of the duration of the irradiation one differentiates between two forms of brachytherapy:

▪ *Afterloading (temporary brachytherapy)*: Here the tumour tissue is "spiked" with catheters or cannulas in a short invasive procedure. Alternatively the applicator is placed in already existing body cavities (e.g. in the case of gynaecological tumours) through which the radiation source is later applied to the tumour. Normally the irradiation lasts for three to five minutes. Three to five afterloading irradiations are usually required.

Afterloading therapy is *widely applied*, frequently with gynaecological tumours, tumours in the ENT area, metastases as well as bronchial, oesophagus, prostate, mammary and floor of mouth carcinomas. Afterloading brachytherapy is often combined with external irradiation or chemotherapy.

- *Seed implantation (permanent brachytherapy)*: In seed implantation implants (seeds) of roughly 4.5 millimetres are implanted into the tumour to destroy it from the inside using palladium or iodine isotopes (type of atom). The implants themselves have a very low dose rate.

I wasn't aware of brachytherapy at the time of my therapy research and did therefore not consider it. By now I know numerous patients who are having their metastases successfully eliminated through afterloading. As this therapy generally only necessitates a brief hospitalisation and the procedure itself is not too strenuous, the patient's quality of life is not overly affected. If distant metastasis of ACC is treated with chemotherapy, the median survival after diagnosis has shown to be circa 13.8 months.

Neutron therapy

For the sake of completeness I also have to mention neutron therapy. Neutron radiation is an ionising radiation consisting of free neutrons. The initially very high expectations in cancer treatment with neutron radiation could not be met, however. Neutrons release the major part of their dosage on the surface and present therefore an extremely limited area of application. It is increasingly less offered by radiotherapy clinics.

In Europe neutron therapy was pioneered in England. Today it is no longer allowed in that country. In the United States only two of the original twelve clinics still exist. In Germany, too, neutron therapy has been severely reduced. An example is the Deutsche Krebsforschungszentrum (the German Cancer Research Centre) in Heidelberg which has discontinued neutron therapy treatment.

For that reason I did not consider this type of radiotherapy.

Protons and carbon ions

Particle radiation with protons and carbon ions is nowadays superior in many respects to photon radiation which is mainly employed in oncological radiotherapy. As this kind of radiotherapy is still relatively rare and as such also largely unknown in professional circles, I shall address it comprehensively in this chapter.

Particle radiation is most effective where the beam is stopped. At this point, the Bragg peak, the tumour tissue absorbs the highest single dose.

After that there is a rapid dosage drop to almost zero. Medical physicists can determine this position to within the millimetre. This facilitates an extremely accurate tumour irradiation and maximum protection of the healthy surrounding tissue. What's more, carbon ions have such a high biological effectiveness that they can also be used to fight tumours where conventional radiotherapy (e.g. photons) is powerless.

Figure 1 shows a comparison of dosage distribution between the three types of radiation: photons, protons and carbon ions *in front of*, *in* and *behind* the tumour. Radiation therapists aim to introduce a maximum dose of the damag-

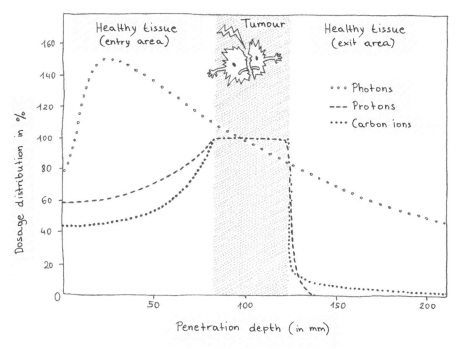

Fig. 1: *Comparative depth dose distribution in the irradiation of tumour tissue with photons, protons and carbon ions.*
[www.teilchen.at/kdm/17]

ing radiation into the tumour tissue while simultaneously protecting the healthy tissue as much as possible. This works very well for radiation with protons or carbon ions and the maximum dosage is inside the tumour.

Photon radiation, however, already develops its maximum dosage after a short penetration depth. In the case of a deep tumour only a reduced amount of the dose can thus contribute to its destruction. The high dose of photon radiation in the radiation entry area can cause serious damage in conjunction with side effects. In practice it is therefore generally attempted to mitigate the problem through irradiation from several angles.

What constitutes the "anti-cancer ammunition" in particle therapy?

Protons or carbon ions are prepared for the treatment in an ion source. To this end an electron is "stolen" from a hydrogen atom to charge the proton (see Figure 2).

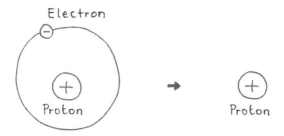

Fig. 2: An electron is "stolen" from a hydrogen atom and only the positively charged proton remains.

A carbon atom, on the other hand, contains six protons and six neutrons in its nucleus plus two electrons in the first outer shell and four electrons in its valence shell (see Figure 3).

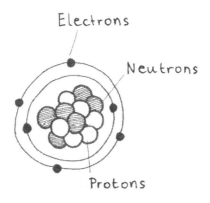

Fig. 3: Carbon atom.

How does a carbon atom become a carbon ion?

Ions are atoms which have either more or less electrons than protons. Because of this imbalance Ions are electrically charged. If one to six electrons are removed from a carbon atom, it turns into a positively charged carbon ion.

When all six electrons are removed we have C12 ions as they consist of six neutrons and six protons.

The carbon ions used in radiation are fully ionised carbon atoms. Thus they now only consist of the carbon atom's nucleus with six protons and six neutrons. As such a carbon

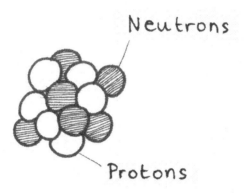

Fig. 4: Carbon ion/C12 ion.

ion is approx. twelve times heavier than a proton and has six times its nuclear charge. In radiotherapy this facilitates a better lateral distribution of the absorbed dose as well as a higher relative biological effectiveness (RBE).

The RBE is mainly based on double-strand breaks of the DNA in the nucleus and is dependent on linear energy transfer (LET), the radiation dose and the irradiated tissue.

A drawback of carbon ion radiotherapy as compared to proton therapy is the fact that immediately *behind* the Bragg peak a small residue of the absorbed dose still meets the healthy tissue. Yet a drawback of proton as opposed to carbon ion radiation is an increased *lateral* distribution into healthy tissue.

Choosing one or the other of these treatments therefore depends on the type of tumour and its position.

After their preparation in the ion source, the protons or the carbon ions respectively are accelerated to approx. two thirds of the speed of light through a circular accelerator (synchrotron or cyclotron). Due to their mass, the protons and carbon ions form a linear, sharply defined beam with only minimal dispersion and can therefore be very accurately aimed at the tumour. They barely infiltrate healthy tissue and develop their effect predominantly inside their target, the tumour. This protects the surrounding tissue as much as possible and the dose inside the tumour can be significantly increased. It also increases the probability of fully destroying the tumour and healing the patient. Furthermore, carbon ions also affect metabolically less active cells, which practically exist in every tumour, as well as tumours with weak blood circulation and low in oxygen and slowly growing tumours. Compared to protons, carbon ions are on average three times more biologically effective. This means the likelihood of irreparable cell damage can be multiplied with carbon ions as compared to protons and photos while using the same radiation dose.

Consequently even tumours which can rarely be treated with conventional radiotherapy or proton radiation can be irradiated with carbon ions with good results.

The advantage of low lateral dispersion during carbon ion treatment is important for my kind of tumour, which is located very close to the brain, as the brain is less affected.

At this point I would like to mention that there are also less

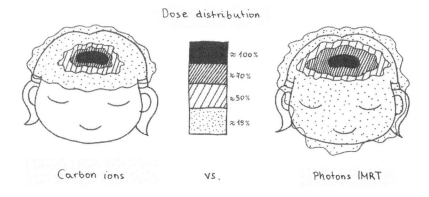

Fig. 5: Comparison of dose distribution in radiation
treatment: carbon ions versus photons.
[Amaldi & Kraft (2005); Ellerbrock (2009)]

radiation-resistant tumours than mine which could absolutely be treated with photon radiation. The advantages hereby are that most hospitals offer it, that it is less expensive and more tolerant regarding unsteadiness, body movements through breathing or changes in the body through fluctuating weight. In my case, however, based on the low tumour control rate, photon irradiation could definitely be ruled out.

Figure 5 shows a graphically simplified comparison of two treatment plans for a brain tumour. Irradiation with carbon ions on the left (two beam directions) and on the right irradiation with photons IMRT (nine beam directions).

The comparison illustrates that during particle radiation with carbon ions the radiation dose can be very well adjusted to the tumour and only very little of the healthy tissue is also irradiated. This is similar during particle radiation with protons.

With photon radiation, however, even though nine different beam directions are utilised (IMRT) to evenly distribute the high dose, healthy tissue is more widely affected.

This happens because the photon beams already emit a large part of their energy on their way to the tumour, but also afterwards into surrounding healthy tissue. This increases the probability of side effects. Repeat irradiation of possible future recurrences in the also exposed healthy tissue may have to be forfeited as well.

These facts made me increasingly suspect that particle radiation with carbon ions or protons would probably be my best option.

What is the success rate of treating tumours with carbon ions?

As early as 1994 the National Institute of Radiological Sciences (NIRS) in Japan started to research the effectiveness of carbon ions in the treatment of a large number of different tumours.

A high local tumour control rate has confirmed the advantages of the biological and physical properties of carbon ion irradiation for nearly all types of tumours. Carbon ion beams are high linear energy transfer (LET) beams whose energy output steadily increases from its entry point into the body at greater depth and reaches its maximum dose in the more deep-seated tumour shortly before it comes to a stop (Bragg peak). In Japan, head and neck tumours of the cranial base and the upper cervical spine, non-small cell lung cancer, hepatocellular carcinoma (liver cancer), prostate cancer, bone and soft tissue sarcomas, cervical, rectal and pancreatic cancer as well as eye tumours are treated specifically, with excellent results in some instances. At this stage scientists even suspect that carbon ion therapy may prevent metastatic spread, for example through the double-strand breaks in the tumour cell's DNA. If this hypothesis is confirmed it would no doubt be another milestone in medical cancer research. [Tsujii & Kamada (2012); Tsujii, Mizoe, Kamada et al. (2007); Akino, Teshima, Kihara et al. (2009)]

The knowledge about the NIRS radiotherapy centre's successes I had acquired during my research had now ultimately convinced me to select a carbon ion therapy for the treatment of my disease (ACC).

I was aware that it would be extremely difficult to be accepted as a patient because only two countries worldwide offered irradiation with carbon ions: Germany and Japan.

I therefore seriously considered irradiation with protons as a second option.

But first I had to establish if my type of tumour, the adenoid cystic carcinoma (ACC), even qualified for either proton or carbon ion therapy.

What type of tumours can be irradiated with protons or carbon ions?

My research showed that a tumour must have the following characteristics to have a chance of being treated with protons or carbon ions:

- The tumour is malignant.
- The tumour is reasonably segregated from other tissue.
- Surgery is difficult or impossible.
- The tumour is radiation-resistant to other types of radiation and therefore requires a very high dose which cannot be achieved with other radiotherapies.
- The tumour does not yet metastasise (in rare cases metastases are also irradiated).
- There must be no metal present in the area to be irra-

diated. If metal has been implanted during previous surgery, carbon ion or proton treatment is no longer an option for this particular area.

■ No pre-irradiation should have been applied to the area in question as otherwise the maximum dose is quickly exceeded.

My salivary gland cancer in the parotid, the adenoid cystic carcinoma (ACC), fulfilled all these criteria.

Specifically the following tumours are currently irradiated with protons or carbon ions - in some instances very successfully - in various clinics around the world. Due to those clinics' different fields of specialisation not every type of tumour is treated in each of them.

■ Tumours in the head and neck area
■ Brain and skull base tumours
■ Eye tumours
■ Lung and liver tumours
■ Tumours in the abdomen and pelvic area
■ Prostate carcinomas
■ Rectal cancer
■ Tumours and metastases in the spine area
■ Breast tumours * (in clinical trials with carbon ions)
■ Pancreatic carcinomas
■ Chordomas and chondrosarcomas (bone tumours) of the skull base
■ Chordomas and chondrosarcomas (bone tumours) of the pelvis
■ Soft tissue sarcomas
■ Pediatric tumours
■ In special cases also local recurrences and metastases

Not treatable are:
■ Itinerant tumours such as those of the upper colon or leukaemia
■ Tissue previously irradiated with high dosages

*News to me was that breast tumours (stage 1) are also irradiated with carbon ions in clinical trials in Japan. For a long time the breast lumps' mobility had made it impossible to irradiate them accurately. Meanwhile the problem has been solved. Since 2013 small isolated Stage 1 tumours are being irradiated with carbon ions in clinical trials in Japan. From 2017 on, irradiating breast tumours with carbon ions is intended to be included in the standard programme. [Interview with my attending radiation expert in Japan, Dr Hasegawa, on 12.07.2015 in Vienna]

Generally the same area can only be irradiated once with protons or carbon ions (circa 70 Gray max.). Patients who have previously been treated with other types of radiation will presumably not be accepted as renewed irradiation would exceed the highest possible total radiation dose for the tissue. This could result in the formation of unmanageable necrosis which can become life- threatening especially if located in the brain.

One dosage unit of radiotherapy is called a Gray (abbreviated to Gy) and specifies how much energy is absorbed by the tissue. The required dose to destroy the tumour is determined by its radiation sensitivity and ranges between 20 to 70 Gy. Individual radiation types also differ in terms of their biological efficacy. This is referred to as *relative biological effectiveness (RBE)*. It is defined as the ratio of an energy dose of a radiation (e.g. photons) to a reference radiation. Compared to photons, protons have a 1.1 higher biological effectiveness. That of Carbon ions is even two to four times higher than that of photons.

To keep side effects to a minimum, the total dose is usually divided into smaller individual doses. As the adenoid cystic carcinoma is very resistant to radiation, I was given 16 x 4 Gy, i.e. 64 Gy in total. The more Gy are required to destroy a tumour the more important it is to choose a radiation type which targets it as accurately as possible with the least damage to surrounding tissue.

NECROSIS - death of tissue OR AN ORGAN.

How to find the right radiation clinic

Many clinics specialise in the treatment of specific types of tumours. I therefore recommend also sending your medical records to institutions outside your own country and to enquire if and how the appropriate treatment for your symptoms would be conducted. Personally I visited three radiation clinics until I felt certain that I'd found "the right one". By now there is a relatively large number of proton radiation treatment centres in countries including Germany, England, France, Italy, Poland, Sweden, the Czech Republic, Switzerland, Austria, Canada, the USA, South Africa, China, Japan, South Korea and Taiwan.

As of 2010, clinics using carbon ion radiation only existed in Germany and Japan. At this stage such facilities are also available in Italy, China and, since 2017/2018, in Austria. For an overview of all particle therapy facilities visit the Particle Therapy Co-operative Group's website at *www.ptcog.ch/index.php/facilities-in-operation.*

Visiting various radiation clinics begins...

Munich

In 2010 no therapy facilities for my particular type of tumour existed in Austria which met my standards. I therefore first considered the proton therapy centre in Munich, not least because of its geographical proximity.

We established contact by phone and forwarded all the necessary records and a current MRI image. More or less patiently I then waited an entire month because I was under the impression that such a large radiation centre would have to deal with quite a lot of enquiries. Their website, too, suggested an enormous workload. But after I still hadn't heard back over a month later and had suspected a speedy response wouldn't be forthcoming, I rang again to ask if they might possibly need additional documentation to finally at least be granted an appointment. I was subsequently informed that even a first consultation required a financial commitment for the complete treatment cost.

I would have been able to pay this through my national health insurance. But this may have entailed even further delays or even a refusal. Or I could have paid for it out of my own pocket, as they informed me. After I'd quickly noticed that money played a major part, I asked them what kind of fees would be involved. They named a sum and I agreed to transfer the funds - which would have bought an average-priced car - but I was luckily in a position to borrow the money. At the time I found their charges utterly excessive as I was only looking for a first consultation. But I realised that the centre wanted to safeguard its interests in advance in view of the already tangible treatment.

Early December 2010, my mother and I drove to Munich for the long anticipated initial consultation and to determine the further strategy for possible proton radiation. Secretly I hoped to have found the right place at last and to start my therapy straight away. Thus I arrived with a packed suitcase, confident and extremely motivated, expecting to stay in the clinic for quite some time. We moved into a double room in the adjacent guesthouse. In the evening we discussed what to do so we wouldn't get lost in the hustle and bustle of the clinic's expected hectic daily routine.

The following morning we headed for the clinic's main wing. I nearly felt like being on the threshold of a personal historic moment. The so eagerly anticipated consultation, the start of being liberated from my torment was just moments away. We stepped into the building expecting a fully booked clinic and paused in reverence. What we saw, however, was a large, deserted hall where merely two lonely patients wandered along the empty corridors. The only audible sounds were our own footsteps. We stared at each other, slightly disconcerted by the realisation that this unexpected scene surprised us equally. After a few deep breaths I asked myself how it could have taken more than a month to secure an appointment in this place. Initially I still believed there had been some kind of error and that we would be engulfed by busy activity as soon as we turned around the next corner. With growing bewilderment I then realised that in this part of the just opened building at least life consisted mainly of the two of us.

My astonishment would, however, soon after be surpassed by bitter disappointment once we had found the correct floor and room. Just two minutes into the long awaited consultation session I was emphatically advised to have surgery first and then radiotherapy. In their view, the physicians explained, the chances of successful radiotherapy were the bigger the less tumour tissue was still present. But this was just the type of procedure I didn't want. I was still adamant that I had to avoid surgery at all costs!

Looking back today I know that the physical dose distribution of protons is clearly superior to the dose distribution of conventional photon beams and thus introduces a higher dose into the target area (the tumour) while simultaneously being easy on the surrounding healthy/normal tissue. Proton beams do, however, develop a similar biological effectiveness to those of photons (RBE = 1.1). Thus DNA damage to the tumour cells in an ACC tumour would have been little more effective than photon radiation. I am therefore now glad that I had been refused back then, as proton treatment for ACC without surgery would have entailed a high probability of recurrence.

Having said this, other slightly more radiosensitive tumours (e.g. prostate carcinomas) are now successfully irradiated with protons, even without surgery.

At the time we went home deeply disappointed. Besides we had also lost an entire month through the long wait for an appointment in Munich. Valuable time when my facial nerve paralysis had significantly progressed through the tumour's growth. As expected, the clinic returned my down payment less a small consultation fee. I now hope that in future patients don't have to pay a deposit amounting to half the full therapy costs for just the initial consultation or that a health insurance company has to vouch for covering the costs. Neither the administrative nor the medical staff of a clinic should ever be obliged to delay possibly urgent treatment.

Heidelberg

After radiotherapy in Munich with prior surgery was out of the question for me we started looking for alternatives. Through extensive research in medical journals besides other sources and direct contact with the university hospital in Heidelberg we found that my type of tumour (ACC) could probably be irradiated in Germany even without prior surgery. So our next destination was Heidelberg.

At my interview at the radiology department in Heidelberg one of the physicians explained the radiation procedure and that they would irradiate the affected side of my face, my neck and with that also the lymph. The physician handed me a fact sheet outlining all the details as well as some of the side effects. Over the course of my research I had read about far more side effects than listed in the leaflet. When I told the physician so she admitted to additional ones such as skin burns, dysphagia (discomfort in swallowing), xerostomia (dry mouth), deafness and tinnitus.

On the one hand I was glad to have found a clinic that would use radiotherapy without surgery in the treatment of my tumour, on the other I saw myself faced with a multitude of undesirable side effects. Presumably like most patients I started hoping that they wouldn't be so bad after all. Although the possibility of side effects was pointed out, it was not mentioned that they would most probably occur, as I knew from my research.

Overall the consultation was quite comprehensive and confirmed my hope of beating the disease without surgical intervention. I was asked if I knew the exact type of my tumour as the therapy in Heidelberg differentiated the total area to be irradiated depending on the carcinoma, i.e. adenocarcinoma or adenoid cystic carcinoma.

Even if small there was still some hope that my case "only" entailed an adenocarcinoma. This would have meant that the lymph wouldn't also have to be irradiated and a smaller radiation field would have to be targeted. As the specialist mentioned highly probable skin changes due to the radiation - which I naturally wanted to avoid at all costs - it seemed expedient to have another histology (tissue analysis) performed in Vienna.

> Today I know that there are radiotherapies where it is irrelevant what exact tumour subtypes are involved. In retrospect this additional histology only served statistical purposes. I regret having had it performed.

While taking our leave, still shaking hands, I asked if I would receive a treatment appointment at the earliest possible opportunity after the still to be conducted histological analysis in Vienna and the precise tumour classification. This was important to me because I had read that it was advisable not to wait too long between surgery and the subsequent radiotherapy. But it is also important that surgical wounds have healed properly before radiation treatment. To prevent too great an interval I therefore tried to establish as precisely as possible when my radiotherapy could start. That way I could have the histology test shortly before.

The specialist reassured me that there would be no delay and a place would be available forthwith. This made me rejoice as my ENT physician in Vienna had offered to carry out the procedure to establish the exact type of tumour the following week. "Yes, that's perfect timing!" I was told. "Do it next week and call us once the wound has healed so we can book you in!"

I liked the fact that I was just charged a normal consultation fee. Unlike the clinic in Munich which had demanded a substantial deposit. To avoid any more delays I applied to my national health insurance to cover the costs. My request was approved within days.

Inevitable certainty
–
torn between agony and hope

Back home I immediately made an appointment at the out-patient department for ear, nose and throat diseases at the Vienna General Hospital. Here a team removed eight tissue samples under local anaesthetic. The procedure was quite stressful as the individual samples, which had been sent straight to pathology for analysis immediately on extraction, contained no cancer cells whatsoever. The doctor really did his best, but couldn't detect any tumour tissue and unceremoniously closed the incision after the eighth sample. His only explanation was that the tumour must be located deeper in the tissue. And so I was offered another appointment for six days later during the week before Christmas. This time the procedure was performed under general anaesthetic and the removal of four further tissue samples finally produced a clear result. I definitely had an adenoid cystic carcinoma (ACC) and therefore the type which is more extensively irradiated in Heidelberg. My mother and my partner were waiting outside the operating theatre where my otolaryngol-ogist, who had performed the biopsy, presented them with the news. The surgery had taken two and a half hours. My physician considered it a success because he had now found the exact type of malignant cells: an ACC, the more malignant form of salivary gland cancer.

For my mother the certainty initially destroyed all her hopes that everything would be alright. Later I learned that she broke down in tears when the doctor gave her the diagnosis. Helplessly he stood beside her and asked what she could possibly have expected. Should she have told him that a mother hopes and prays until the very end that everything is just a bad dream? He then assured her: "You will feel better once your daughter is being treated." And he was right, as it turned out, but we still had a long way to go before the right therapy. Still sitting in the hospital's corridor she asked him: "Does my daughter already know?" He nodded. My mother and my partner immediately wanted to join me in the recovery room to support me when I had to deal with the terrible verdict. But as I was already 28 years old, they couldn't. Parents are only allowed in recovery until their child is 18; boyfriends and partners not at all. My mother was completely beside herself when she couldn't be with me. My partner was also on the verge of tears. But despite the terrible diagnosis he remained optimistic and told her with confidence: "I know that everything will be fine." A wonderfully positive thought which greatly boosted my mental strength and convalescence.

Now having a definite diagnosis, I wanted to agree a radiotherapy appointment with the clinic in Heidelberg. Instead I was met with a rude awakening. The verbal commitment to a speedy treatment was forgotten. I now would have to wait for more than two months for a new appointment where I would receive 25 x 2 Gy of photons and 8 x 3 Gy of carbon ions. When my mother pleaded with them for an earlier date, they suggested an exclusive photon therapy as an alternative.

Luckily, through our research, we already knew at the time that patients with ACC are only offered an exclusive photon IMRT if carbon ion therapy is not readily available.

Regarding the tumour control rate (this expresses the probability of a tumour's non-continuing growth in percent), a comparative study states that exclusive photon radiotherapy merely reaches a control rate of 24.6 percent, four years after treatment. A control rate of 77.5 percent, however, is reported for a beam combination of photons and carbon ions.

I also read in Wannemacher, Debus and Wenz's book "Strahlentherapie" ("Radiotherapy"): "A randomised phase III study comparing a combination therapy with carbon ion boost to an exclusive photon IMRT would therefore not be ethically feasible." [Wannemacher, Debus & Wenz (2006): p. 169: Maligne Speicheldrüsentumoren (Malign Salivary Gland Tumours)]

So, for timing reasons, I was offered a radiation treatment which promised very little chance of recovery for my type of tumour. A treatment which already years before had been deemed as physically inferior when compared to a carbon ion combination therapy and as ethically not feasible.

My research had saved me from the grave consequences of agreeing to the wrong treatment. As the same tumour can only be irradiated once, the wrong decision would have been fatal. A 75.4 percent probability of recurrence in the case of ACC is definitely life-threatening. Searching for a plausible explanation I discovered there are shortages in the availability of carbon ions. Back then they were only available for irradiation in Japan and Germany, and that certain irradiation cycles evidently exist.

The patients' radiotherapy starts at a set date, more or less simultaneously, and takes place within a specific period in accordance with a strict schedule. An individual patient being treated outside this schedule is therefore hardly possible.

My suspicion was later confirmed in Japan and so I reckon that other clinics proceed in the same way. I urgently recommend planning a possible treatment and arranging appointments as quickly as possible.

Christmas 2010

For quite some time my family and I had wished to take a city break in New York and combine it with the New Year's Eve celebrations in Times Square. This year we meant to fulfil our dream and fly to the Big Apple for Christmas and New Year.

The flights had been booked long before my cancer diagnosis and until a few weeks before our departure I was still determined to go. But at Christmas I suddenly lost heart. It was Christmas Eve before the stitches from my last biopsy were removed and my hair was so greasy after not having been washed for ages (so as not to compromise the healing process), it practically shone as brightly as the Christmas tree.

I didn't feel comfortable. What if there were sudden complications after all? What if I developed pain?

Many questions and emotions occupied me that Christmas Eve – a time usually associated with joyful anticipation and radiant faces. Instead there were tears rolling down my cheeks.

Would I ever spend Christmas with my family again without being in pain? Would I be in hospital next Christmas? How would my facial paralysis develop? Would the cancer get out of hand and beat me?

Devastation – what now?

My siblings flew to New York as planned. But my mother no longer felt in the mood for a holiday and so gladly stayed in Vienna with me when I asked her. I was relieved. Had she been thousands of miles away in a medical emergency, I would have felt terribly helpless. Nobody knows more about my medical history than my mother after all. And hardly anyone is as tenacious as my mother when it comes to representing my interests. After I had spontaneously decided to visit my partner's family in Germany, my mother stayed behind in Vienna. Which quite suited her as she had planned to keep trying for an earlier appointment in Heidelberg and to step up her research into my disease.

I had read that radiotherapy patients in Heidelberg lost about 45 pounds on average. So I decided to stop dieting. At that stage I weighed just under eight stone because I had tried retarding the cancer's growth by changing to a diet low in carbohydrates and sugars. But now I had reached a point where I told myself "It's enough! Start eating again. You have to eat! You don't want to be fed through a nasal or gastric tube if the treatment damages your mucous membranes so much you can no longer swallow." So I planned to put on some "just in case" weight. I used the Christmas period to stuff myself, particularly with lots of biscuits. During advent I had baked enormous amounts of them without even tasting the tiniest morsel myself.

The first ray of hope

Not willing to give up, my mother consulted another physician over the Christmas period – a practitioner specialising in nuclear medicine recommended by a friend of hers – to discuss the situation and explore further alternatives. This subsequently led to contacting a Japanese doctor, an accredited radiation oncology specialist, who worked in the field of tumour treatment. The connection to Japan was quickly established despite the festive season. He offered his help and asked for the latest MRI results to be emailed. On receipt he instantly analysed them and reported back just a day later. He was the first medical professional to categorise the size of my tumour as relatively small and did not foresee any problems regarding the treatment. Moreover, he imme-diately made it clear that he would exclusively irradiate the growth with carbon ions. This very much corresponded to my wishes, as our extensive research had distinctly shown that carbon ion therapy represented the very best of all treat-ment options for my type of cancer.

The specialist envisaged a 96 percent probability of re-covery. During a subsequent, personal consultation he even mentioned 98 percent due to the tumour's still relatively small size and the fact that it had not previously been oper-ated on. I was overwhelmed!

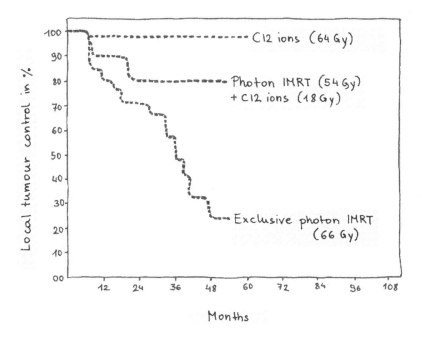

Fig. 6: Probability of local tumour control through exclu-sive carbon ion (C12) irradiation, compared to an combi-nation of photon IMRT + C12 and to an exclusive photon IMRT, when applied to ACC.
[Schulz-Ertner, Nikoghosyan, Didinger et al. (2005)]

Figure 6 illustrates this – if quite simple – as a line showing the best predicted result, even after five years (60 months), i.e. a local tumour control rate of 96 percent (stages T1-T3) if an ACC tumour in the head and neck region is treated with an exclusive carbon ion therapy. For me this line symbolises healing.

To understand the overwhelming happiness I felt when thinking about the treatment, one has to remember those therapies which only produced a probable tumour control rate of 24.6 percent for my type of tumour four years after photon IMRT (66 Gy) irradiation and 77.5 percent after combined irradiation with photon IMRT (54 Gy) and carbon ions (18 Gy) (see Figure 6).

It clearly shows how vastly local tumour control rates vary with different radiotherapies and that survival may depend on the type of treatment.

Later I also had a closer look at figures regarding the success rates of carbon ion treatment for other tumour types and was impressed with the NIRS's achievements in Japan.

A high local irradiation dose of carbon ion can also damage the DNA of slow-growing, usually well regenerating tumour cells to such an extent that they're generally unable to further reproduce themselves. This stops the tumour's growth. In many instances the tumour cell then activates its own suicide programme and dies (apoptosis).

The choice of radiotherapy does not only affect local tumour control rates, but also the probability of developing metastases differs depending on the chosen treatment.

Impressively, only 14% of patients developed metastases after combined irradiation with photons and carbon ions, whilst 68% of patients developed metastases within 4 years after photon irradiation (see Table 1).

You may ask: Why is the risk of getting metastases after been irradiated with carbon-ion and photons much lower compared being irradiated with photons only?

67

Number of patients	Treatment	Number of patients with metastases	in %
34	Photons	23 (4 years)	68
29	Photons + C-ion	4 (4 year)	14

Table 1: Metastatic potential of combined irradiation compared to photon radiation only (for adenoid cystic carcinomas – ACC).

Carbon-ion radiotherapy induces the so-called immunogenetic cell death. The immunogenetic cell death might act as an in situ "tumour vaccine" and initiate an important immune response. This immune reaction generates antigens which stimulate T-cells to become cytotoxic T-cells. These cytotoxic T-cells are supposed to attack cancer cells including micrometastases and circulating tumour cells. Therefore, C-ion radiotherapy might induce tumour regression even of nonirradiated tumours (called abscopal effect). Carbon ion even suppresses the metastatic potential when irradiated with a lower, sublethal dose. Photon irradiation, on the other hand, increases the metastatic potential when irradiated with a sublethal dose. Moreover, photon radiation at a lower dose might acquire a more aggressive phenotype of metastases. Therefore, radiation fields and dosage have to be carefully determined also from this point of view.

The doors to an extremely interesting alternative had now opened up for me. But it was still incredibly far away. I had still planned on going to Heidelberg after having resigned myself to wait for the treatment. The important preparations were more or less finished and I had long since invested all my hope in being cured there. The sudden thought of changing to another clinic made me feel uneasy. For months I'd had to make concrete and right decisions and to go back on them now entailed a certain amount of insecurity. I even asked myself if it would be the right thing to do. Besides, I was extremely scared to be rejected in Japan, just as I had been in Munich and over the phone by a clinic in Boston, because I had definitely ruled out prior surgery. What's more, for the time being my national health insurers could not confirm that they would cover the costs because they had only just approved the treatment in Heidelberg. I was therefore facing the additional risk of temporarily having to pay for the therapy myself. All these factors intensified my inner conflict and helplessness until my mother finally convinced me with the words: "Nina, a lot of people nowadays go on exotic holidays, so let's just think of it as a break!"

The idea of simply viewing my trip to Japan as a holiday if they refused to treat me there was an ingenious ploy to soothe my frayed nerves. Secretly I wondered how often I would still be able to travel. So even if Japan proved to be a disappointment, I would at least have seen the country and bridged the long wait for the treatment in Heidelberg at the same time! My mother had already been in touch with the attending physicians in the Far East and they were convinced that the chances of successful treatment were promising.

I decided to risk going on the journey.

Hopeful journey to Japan

I was now facing the small challenge of finding out how to best protect myself from possible side effects during radiotherapy. My mother actively supported me in the endeavour. We found various radiotherapy self-help groups on the internet. Based on their recommendations we eventually flew to Japan armed with a whole suitcase full of crèmes, oils, mouthwashes and other personal care products. We had been advised not to use products containing zinc because it diverts the beams and can therefore obstruct targeted irradiation. Some of the products we brought turned out to be extremely helpful later on.

Amongst other things we packed:

- a tea blend of nettles, wild mallow leaves and bay leaves
- sage tea (also supposed to counteract stomatitis – inflammation of the mouth's mucous membrane)
- mouthwashes for inflamed mucous membranes
- artificial saliva from the chemist
- an inhaler in case of a cold, including saline solution and a suitable cough expectorant

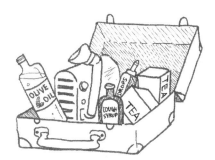

- cough syrup, cough-relieving tea and cough drops
- olive oil
- St. John's wort oil
- antiseptic ointments
- cortisone cream
- pH strips
- globules to counteract radiation damage (radium bromide C30)

At the beginning of January we boarded our plane and were lucky to be seated in a row with ample legroom. But our joy was short-lived when a noisy German-speaking tour group positioned itself right in front of us. After a while, however, listening in to their chatter was funny enough to make us more relaxed and nearly feel like being on holiday. Time proverbially flew by.

Arriving in Japan

Once arriving in Japan we showed a taxi driver a note with the address of our lodgings. Like his colleagues he just shrugged his shoulders and we would presumably still be stranded outside the airport if we hadn't had the foresight to also have our temporary address translated into Japanese characters.

The apartment that the clinic had organised for us in advance was typically Japanese: just a very small living space with a kitchenette and a tiny adjacent wet room with a sit-only bathtub and no heating. The toilet's cistern featured an integrated sink. The water flowed from the sink into the toilet, thus serving the dual function of washing your hands and flushing the toilet with the same water.

The tiny hall led into a small living room and from there into a bedroom, divided by sliding doors, which just about accommodated two single beds. This was handy enough because we could actually watch the TV in the living room from our beds. The living room featured a heating carpet (an electric carpet that heats) and wall-mounted air-conditioning.

One night my mother accidentally entered the wrong remote control commands for the air-conditioning and the heating went on strike. The room temperature rapidly dropped from roughly 22 °C to 15 °C.

Slightly panicking in view of the snow outside we randomly pressed some more buttons. Of course, they were all labelled in Japanese. Miraculously the heating started working again and the temperature went back up to a blissful 22 degrees.

In January it's about as cold in Japan as it is back home in Austria, roughly zero degrees and snowing. My mother insisted we immediately buy a radiator for the hall. She worried that my treatment could be jeopardised if I caught a cold.

So we went to the nearby shopping centre in search of a heater and something to eat.

The range of products in the supermarket was overwhelming. Never before had I seen such a large assortment of low-priced, freshly caught fish, sushi, meat, vegetables, fruit and pastries. Everything was prepared for sale in a separate room right behind the serving counters. Sushi and makizushi, too, were freshly made every hour and whatever wasn't sold within three hours was then offered at half price. The fish dishes were so fresh, I started quipping that the unsold cut price fish was presumably packaged and exported to Europe.

Equipped with a heater, the best of fish, vegetables and mineral water we headed home for a cosy evening in.

First consultation at the
NIRS treatment centre

Refreshed by some excellent food, we started exploring our immediate surroundings so we'd easily find the clinic the next day.

When we got there we were slightly disappointed that it didn't seem as modern as we had imagined. But seeing that the centre had been established in 1957 it was hardly surprising. Nonetheless it had greatly influenced worldwide research and development, diagnosis and treatment in radiological applications for the past decades. As early as 1994 it started treatment with carbon ions and as such Japan is *the* pioneer in the field of this particular therapy option. Moreover, the NIRS (National Institute of Radiological Sciences) is engaged in the research of side effects as well as the protection from radiation exposure to human health and the environment.

The following day the interpreter who was already expecting us at the clinic, explained the general concept of a treatment contract. During the subsequent consultation a medical specialist went over *my* contract with us in detail and in English. He also outlined the probability of potential short- and long-term side effects I might develop.

Particularly reassuring was that the clinic's medical director guaranteed me a 98 percent probable tumour control rate for five years. My chances of success, he elaborated, were so positive because my tumour was relatively small and had not previously been operated on.

The lymph nodes in my neck would not be irradiated as they weren't affected according to the MRI. This differed from the treatment plans of the other clinics I had visited and corresponded exactly to my wishes.

It also made sense to me. Why irradiate something that's presumably cancer-free? Should an affected lymph node show up on an MRI at a later stage, it could be irradiated or removed at the time. Preventative irradiation would deprive me of renewed radiotherapy if a tumour appeared in the already treated area.

He also told me that the last two biopsies that had been performed in Vienna were irrelevant when it came to the exact classification of my tumour because both possible types, i.e. an adenocarcinoma or an adenoid cystic carcinoma, are irradiated in the same way.

Those two biopsies, which turned out to be unnecessary in retrospect, are the only decisions I regret. Apart from the medical irrelevance, I now have scars right around the earlobe which, although small, have left unpleasant nerve injuries.

When I asked the Japanese specialist if my facial nerve would recover, he replied: "Unfortunately no." Disappointed, I checked: "Is there really no chance?" He said no again.

I didn't want to give up on my dream and have been known to be obstinate at times. So I enquired if there was at least the tiniest possibility of nerve regeneration. He took a deep breath and evidently didn't want to entirely destroy my hopes when he said: "Well, perhaps there's a one percent chance!"

There are two reasons why the probability of regeneration was so low:

- the tumour had infiltrated the nerve and
- it is the more unlikely that a nerve will recover the longer the paralysis has already been present.

This underlines the enormous importance of quickly finding the right treatment to contain damages caused by a tumour as much as possible – not to mention the fact that one's very survival and quality of life depends on it.

Possible side effects of carbon ion treatment in my case

I was handed a detailed list of possible side effects that could occur in my particular case. The short-term ones would most probably include burning of the skin as well as a sensation of weakness in the arms through minor irradiation of the adjacent brain, nausea, tinnitus, ear infection, dry mouth and muscle stiffness.

Possible long-term side effects were also comprehensively explained to me. These are reactions to the irradiation which only present months or years after therapy. But they, too, can frequently be eradicated through suitable treatment.

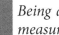 *Being aware of possible side effects facilitates pre-emptive measures to prevent their occurrence to a certain degree.*

Muscles in the irradiated area harden significantly later and thus pose the risk of mobility impairment. To counteract this I exercised my muscles at the start of my treatment to limit the damage as much as possible. Bones in the irradiated area can also tend to become more brittle and have to be surgically replaced in extreme cases. Knowing this made me try everything possible to boost my bone density (see "The importance of a proper diet and dietary supplements", p. 101 et seq.).

When the brain is also irradiated it can lead to damages which can affect the whole body.

In rare cases a secondary tumour can be caused by the radiotherapy ten to twenty years after treatment. In my opinion it is therefore particularly important to counteract this eventuality through a series of anticarcinogenic dietary supplements.

Preparing for the therapy

Following the extensive consultation with the doctor, I received a schedule with an exact list of all my appointments for the preliminary examinations.

Over the next days I had an MRI, a CAT scan, a PET scan and an ENT assessment. These preliminary examinations were included in the flat rate for the radiotherapy.

Based on the results, the doctors prepared a face mask. For this they placed a pleasantly warm and soft but foul-smelling plastic mesh over my face.

Initially it still felt quite loose on my face and shoulder region. But when the fan was switched on the mesh hardened and the mould clung ever more firmly to my facial contours until eventually restricting all freedom of movement, a strange and oppressive feeling. I concentrated on breathing evenly so as not to jeopardise a perfect fit. A mouthpiece, previously specially made in the orthodontic department, served to ease my breathing and simultaneously kept my jaw under the mask firmly fixed in position. This way I could breathe through my nostrils and my mouth. A simple measure which also helps patients who have a cold.

The clinic's staff focused very much on the patients' needs. They would always escort us from one department to the next (MRI, orthodontics, PET, CAT, blood sampling etc.).

This really made us feel well looked after and never helpless. Only some days later, when we were familiar with the clinic's layout, did we walk to the various appointments on our own.

The radiotherapy followed a set schedule. Four successive days of irradiation were followed by three without. This continued for four weeks until I had received 64 Gy in total, 16 treatments of four Gy each.

Radiotherapy procedure

I lay down on the treatment table in the irradiation room, where my body was fixed into position with the face mask and two Velcro straps. Then I was covered with a soft, fluffy blanket to keep me warm. The individual irradiations themselves didn't take very long, about 10 to 15 minutes depending on the position. Each treatment utilised different beam directions for which the patient had to be newly positioned towards the radiation source. The friendly staff repositioned me as not everything was as yet fully-automated in Japan. The classical music in the background not only gave me a sense of the timing involved, it also helped me to relax by imagining scenes like lying down in a meadow, watching butterflies.

The thought that every radiation kills tumour cells made me feel extremely positive and optimistic about the treatment. My mother even experienced moments of happiness while waiting for me outside the radiation room.

As carbon ion irradiation is completely painless, I felt as if absolutely nothing had happened after the first treatment. Slightly worried, I shared this with my mother. There was no redness of the skin and I wondered if the radiation equipment had even been turned on. I received my reply roughly two hours later when I suddenly, out of the blue, developed strong facial pains. Now I knew that something had actually happened during the treatment. I was in no way prepared for the pain and it became so severe that I slumped onto the floor, bawling my eyes out. My mother grabbed me and we somehow managed to get back to the clinic. Fortunately the dispensary was still open and I was immediately given strong painkillers. It took nearly an hour before the pain had completely subsided. Not wanting to suffer like that again, I decided to take prophylactic analgesics right after the next treatment. I naturally enquired why nobody had prepared me for this and provided painkillers in the case of an emergency. The doctors explained that such severe pain is rather uncommon and usually only occurred after several irradiation units, if at all.

After the fourth session I felt able to do without medication. And the pain didn't actually return. Personally I believe that the first treatment destroyed many small nerves which triggered the severe suffering. The pain I experienced at the beginning was pure hell and by far the most torturous experience during the entire healing process. But it also ushered in my wonderful recovery. It was all uphill from here.

What really helped during the therapy

As already mentioned I arrived prepared with a suitcase full of various creams, oils and teas. I tried many of the suggestions recommended in forums and by medical professionals, but only some of them really helped:

- It is important to drink more than enough liquid. I drank **three to four litres every day, particularly:**
  - Water
  - Green tea: I drank a lot of this. We were in Japan, after all, the land of green tea. Only later did I discover that it supposedly makes radiotherapy even more effective and has anticarcinogenic properties.
  - A tea blend of nettles, wild mallow leaves and bay leaves at a ratio of 2:2:1.
    Wild mallow leaves tea ensured that the oral mucosa, which is usually badly affected by irradiation of the head region, could keep regenerating itself and therefore remained balanced. The nettle tea

supported and accelerated the all important detoxification of the body. Its purifying properties have immense significance during irradiation treatment which entails having to dispose of vast amounts of breakdown products. The bay leaves supplement the other two by also purifying the organism.

I recommended drinking large amounts of fluids to other patients who suffered from tiredness and especially nausea. Once they followed the advice, they instantly improved.

- **Cooling the irradiated skin areas.** When my mother burnt her finger two days before my first treatment and immediately tried to cool the area, we thought of cooling my skin after each radiotherapy session as the process also provides some relieve in case of sunburn. So I cooled the irradiated area with frozen drink cans after each treatment. Of course, gel cooling packs are just as suitable. I wrapped the cans in a thin cloth and pressed them to the irradiated area for about 45 minutes. It is important to do this immediately after treatment. From the start I returned to our close-by accommodation to apply cooling to the affected area as soon as possible. Whenever we were delayed at the clinic, my mother would instantly rush over to the nearest vending machine so I could at least apply a cold drinks can. Here it is important to only apply dry cooling so that the treated area doesn't soften and detach itself. One should also only cool at a comfortable temperature and only for as long as one doesn't find it unpleasant.

- **Skin care of the irradiated area:** Using quality olive oil turned out to provide the best skin care for me. But it took some trial and error before I discovered this.

I tried many products, such as a healing ointment which was prescribed in a radiotherapy study I was familiar with, as well as cortisone and various other creams. What I didn't try was baby powder because I wouldn't apply it to sunburn either. None of those creams and ointments helped to soothe my irritated facial skin. Quite the opposite, in fact, I was mostly allergic to them. Once my skin turned so extremely red that I literally had to scrape the cream off just minutes later. It still took several hours until my face changed from being bright red to red, then just red patches until finally returning to normal. It is very important not to use products containing zinc as this ingredient may redirect the beams and thus prevent targeted irradiation. High quality olive oil, which is also available in Japan, did, however, help my skin immensely. I applied it to the affected areas after cooling them.

By following this routine I saw practically no damage to my skin after 16 irradiation units. The doctors were extremely surprised when the highly probable severe skin damage didn't occur. All they found was a slight reddening of the skin as if it had been exposed to the sun for too long.

The therapy was finished at the end of February and after another MRI I flew back to Vienna. We agreed on six-monthly checkups in Europe and sent the follow-up images to Japan for the next five years.

Japan in retrospect

I am often asked tactfully how I feel about my time in Japan. Whenever I think about it, I recall nothing but the best of memories. Apart from the necessary treatment we spent some wonderful and relaxing weeks in this country. It felt nearly like a long holiday. The days simply flew by with walks in the parks and on the nearby beach, with the more or less daily food-shopping, the occasional afternoon nap, e-mailing and internet chats with my partner. Surprisingly we didn't have any English TV channels in our apartment, so we very gladly watched the DVDs we had brought and which we never had the time to watch at home.

I would often have had beautiful dreams about laughing without my facial paralysis and I'd wake up with the feeling of a symmetrical, radiant smile. Although the illusion was shattered as soon as I tried to raise the corners of my mouth symmetrically in front of the mirror, the feeling when waking up was so brilliant that I kept remembering it throughout the day and inevitably had to smile again.

All our fears after reading up on radiotherapies proved to be more or less unfounded. I never felt nauseous, experienced virtually no skin burns, could eat whatever I fancied and had even gained four pounds by the end of the treatment! We had also forged friendships with some Japanese women which we maintain to this day. We were invited to afternoon refreshments and tea ceremonies and were even presented with kimonos! Someday I would like to go back to Japan to thank all the doctors and nurses again and to show them what amazing work they did.

What also impressed me was the way people treated each other, starting with the greeting where everybody bows to each other. Thus people are on the same level right from the outset and always respectful and polite. Back in Vienna I nearly experienced "culture shock" when a shop assistant in a supermarket snapped at me for not being fast enough at the till.

Our stay had made us feel deeply connected with Japan and it's people!

We were therefore all the more devastated by the Fukushima disaster which happened just a week after we'd left Japan.

Right from our arrival we had frequently felt small seismic tremors but initially regarded them as false perceptions induced by jetlag. Once the jetlag disappeared a few days later and the small tremors didn't, however, we realised that they really were minor earthquakes. Now we understood why all the houses were built as earthquake-proof as possible. A little worried, we asked our Japanese friends and were told that a major earthquake strikes the country roughly every 100 years and was already 18 years overdue. My mother joked: "Let's hope it will wait for another four weeks," not suspecting that just a week after returning to Vienna a tsunami would initiate the devastating Fukushima catastrophe.

Fearing that some unforeseen events could prevent my treatment, my mother begged me not to leave our immediate surroundings and always stay close to the clinic. After our return to Vienna we realised how narrowly we had actually avoided the disaster. The major earthquake in Japan had interrupted train connections and roads were no longer passable. Our Japanese friends' letters told us that they had to walk more than 30 miles in the bitter cold to get home from Tokyo the night after the disaster when traffic had come to a standstill. If we, unable to read or speak Japanese, had shared their fate, we would hardly have found our way home. So we were extremely glad that my treatment was finished in time and we could fly home without any complications.

After conventional therapy – personal responsibility continues

According to my physicians, my treatment in Japan had been a success, so I was discharged and flew back to Vienna. As already mentioned, we agreed to send semi-annual MRI images to Japan for assessment.

The suggestion of merely having pictures taken and being torn between hope and fear that the cancer returned made me feel uncomfortable. I know that my kind of cancer tends to recur and to develop metastases. As such just taking MRI images seemed not enough of a preventative measure in my view.

Preventive action to me means actively contributing towards my own wellbeing. I wanted to take my fate into my own hands.

But what could I do? Where should I start? At first I only found references such as: "Just try continuing to live and work the way you did before diagnosis." Statements like that don't make a lot of sense to me because my cancer had presumably been caused by past mistakes that had weakened my immune system. So I made it my goal to find and avoid them in future.

First I asked myself:

What is cancer and how is it caused?

Cancer consists of cells that multiply indefinitely and without consideration for their surroundings. While healthy cells subordinate themselves to the whole organism, cancer cells egotistically fight for their own benefit. They are practically immortal as they can divide without any signs of ageing. Before they divide, they double their genetic material as well as their other cellular components. Two identical daughter cells are generated during the subsequent cell division. The cells can perform this process in the body provided they exist in an optimal environment.

While ordinary cells age and are then led to their pre-programmed death by their genetic make-up (apoptosis), this process is not distinct enough in the cancer cells.

Only once the cancer cells' genetic material is severely damaged does apoptosis also occur in them. This means that everything activating apoptosis in the cancer cells also counteracts the disease.

But what causes cancer in the first place?

Healthy cells divide when new cells of their specific type are needed and stop dividing once enough of them have been generated. The cell lives as long as required and kills itself when its death is necessary. If a cell occasionally "misbehaves" it doesn't yet cause any notable damage to an organism. Genetic mutations, however, can enable a cell to divide and thus multiply when unnecessary.

The formation of additional daughter cells which behave in an antisocial manner leads to the overall order of the organism collapsing with disastrous consequences as the entire body can be damaged by the proliferation of an abnormal cell's clone. So cancer is generated by pathological changes of the DNA's information and therefore mostly acquired during one's lifetime through diseased genetic material. How does this happen?

Even under optimum conditions a healthy body can exhibit cell mutations due to the fundamentally limited accuracy of DNA replication and repair options. Considering the incredible amount of cell divisions during the course of a lifetime and the associated frequent cell mutation, we shouldn't ask ourselves why cancer develops, but rather why it develops relatively seldom.

The answer is simple. In order for a cancer cell to develop from a normal cell several rounds of mutations are necessary, frequently over several decades. As such cancer is more prevalent in old age.

Initially mutated cells don't carry the characteristics of cancer cells. They only develop through repeated mutations and divisions (see Figure 7). Eventually an entirely malignant cell is created which ruthlessly invades foreign tissue. The usually quite prolonged period before the cancer develops gives the body a chance to repair damaged cells or induce apoptosis.

If harmful influences persist, such as the wrong diet, constant stress, feelings of faintness, pollution and first and foremost smoking (which causes approx. 30 percent of all cancer deaths), the immune system is weakened in the long term. This overtaxes endogenous repair mechanisms which can eradicate chromosomal dam-

Cell mutation cycles

Epithelial cells

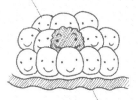

Basal lamina
(Protein layer)

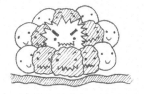

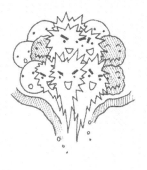

Fig. 7: Mutation and division cycles.

age in the nucleus of healthy cells. The result is permanent cell changes (mutations) which can then generate cancer through further mutations.

It's already apparent that we can often contribute towards preventing the development of cancerous growths by strengthening our immune system. However, the theories that bacteria, fungi or viruses are also contributory cancer causes should, in my view, not be dismissed outright. If it is present in excess, they weaken our immune system which can also lead directly to the damage of a cell's genetic makeup. Similarly cancer can develop if the immune system is weakened through deficiencies (see "'Vitamin B17' – amygdalin – laetrile", p. 149). This needs to be counteracted.

Because each type of cancer develops through a unique combination of mutated genes, it is unlikely that the same treatment works for every patient. Despite the differences, cancer cells also share many commonalities and their associated weaknesses. Tumour cells

1. multiply when restrictions are disregarded and
2. infiltrate tissue reserved for other cells.

When factors 1) and 2) apply, we speak of malignant tumours (cancer). If only factor 1) applies, we speak of benign tumours.

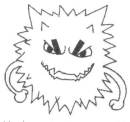

Malignant tumour cell

Malignant tumours can be divided into two major groups: carcinomas and sarcomas. *Carcinomas* are roughly 20 times more common than sarcomas and originate from the epithelial tissue of outer and inner body surfaces. These include the skin and the mucous membrane as well as the linings of glandular organs such as the stomach, the intestines, the breasts, the

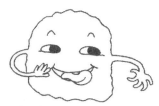

Benign tumour cell

ovaries, the pancreas and the parotid gland. A *sarcoma* is a malignant tumour originating from the mesenchymal cells (connective and supportive tissue). The name is derived from the Greek "Sárka", meaning "flesh", based on the fleshy appearance of soft tissue tumours. Beside malignant tumours like carcinomas and sarcomas there are also malignant tumours of blood-forming organs such as leukaemia, malignant tumours of the central nervous system like glioblastomas or malignant mixed tumours like salivary gland tumours.

Malignant cells can release vascular endothelial growth factors (VEGF) which cause blood vessels to grow in the cell clusters providing the cancer cells with oxygen and nutrients. The formation of new blood vessels in the tumour is called *angioneogenesis* (see Figure 8). Once malignant tumours exceed a size of just a few millimetres, they require their own blood vessels to keep growing. If no new blood vessels are generated, the tumour's growth is inhibited.

Anything which retards angioneogenesis acts as an anti-cancer agent because it impairs the cancer cells' sustenance.

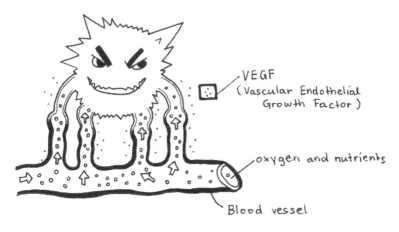

Fig. 8: Angioneogenesis.

But cancer tumours not only grow in healthy tissue, they can also generate secondary tumours (metastases). Here individual cancer cells detach themselves from the original tumour and are transported through the vascular and lymphatic system to other body regions, frequently the liver and the lung, where they settle and survive. Substances that inhibit the cancer cells' ability to settle counteract cancer and the formation of metastases.

Cancer patients mostly don't die from the *primary tumour* (the initial focus of a malignant tumour), but from *metastases* (such as liver, lung and brain metastases).

In summary, it can be said that all substances or treatments which contribute towards

- making the cancer cell commit suicide (apoptosis),
- preventing the formation of new blood vessels in the tumour (angioneogenesis) to impede it from receiving sustenance,
- impairing the cancer cells' ability to settle in other parts of the body (thus counteracting the formation of metastases) and
- making the immune system recognise cancer cells as being alien and therefore treatable

have an anti-cancer effect.

This *makes it clear* that cancer can and has to be fought with several approaches. With orthodox medicine and also much more. As cancer presents with many variations and their associated different attributes, it is expedient to clarify the following questions and base the choice of conventional treatment on the answers:

- Is the tumour fast- or slow-growing?
- Will the tumour respond to chemotherapy?
- Can the tumour be surgically removed in its entirety?
- Is the tumour radiosensitive? (This should determine the type of radiotherapy.)
- Are metastases already present?

- Are there any findings from this particular tumour type having been treated with immunotherapy/antibody therapy?
- Would additional hormone treatment be helpful?

After carefully considered and successfully performed conventional treatment of the tumour, the patient is faced with yet another challenge: preventing the cancer from returning.

Tumour removed – what's next?

Generally cancer can't be "healed" by simply destroying or removing a tumour. In my opinion it expresses a body imbalance far exceeding the actual tumour. Eliminating the tumour is merely the prerequisite for starting the healing process.

Soon after my treatment I therefore consulted a practitioner in complimentary medicine but didn't feel he adequately addressed my questions. He more or less just studied my blood count and concluded it wasn't too bad at all considering I'd just had radiotherapy. I basically didn't have to do anything else! But perhaps I should consider and try mistletoe therapy. And I actually did, but discontinued it eventually because it didn't feel right for me and literally turned me into an insomniac.

How a dream made me change my lifestyle

Not long after, I dreamed about Echinacea. I remembered that even my great-grandmother long ago had always sworn by the plant's beneficial effects on the immune system.

The following day I started reading up on the subject and discovered that taking Echinacea is recommended after radiotherapy to further the renewed growth of leukocytes (white blood cells). A glance at my recent blood tests confirmed that my leukocyte count of 2600/µl was extremely low.

After taking Echinacea on a daily basis for about three weeks it had risen to 3600/µl. At that moment I was sure that I had to actively involve myself in strengthening my immune system for a long-term recovery. My mother and I started searching for solutions to completely prevent the cancer from recurring.

The jigsaw puzzle below is meant to illustrate how I declared war on the disease. My plan was to weaken potentially remaining and newly generated cancer cells from all angles, to eliminate them and give them no chance of returning.

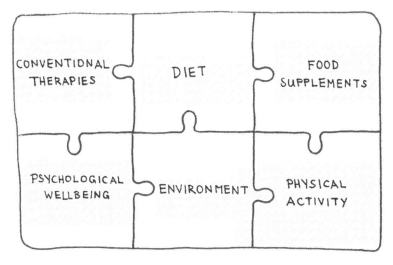

Fig. 9: My anti-cancer jigsaw puzzle.

As the removal of the primary tumour does not necessarily prevent the formation of metastases, which are frequently the cause when cancer results in death. I therefore explored the subject more extensively.

How metastases develop

The formation of metastases is the settlement of migrant cancer cells in other organs where they multiply. Here we differentiate between lymphatic and haematogenous metastasis.

During *lymphatic metastatic spread* the tumour infiltrates lymph vessels which facilitate the tumour cells attaching themselves to the lymph nodes where they multiply. This leads to the generation of lymph node metastases which frequently enter the bloodstream and can form further metastases in other parts of the body.

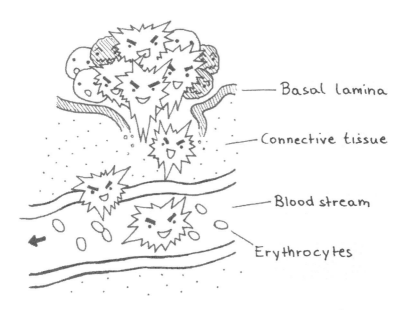

Fig. 10: From the epithelial tissue, the tumour cells of a primary tumour penetrate the basal lamina (protein layer) and reach the vascular or lymphatic system through the connective tissue to settle in other parts of the body (metastasis). [Graw, Alberts, Bray, Hopkin et al. (2012)]

During *haematogenous metastasis* the tumour cells break through the walls of the blood vessels (mostly capillaries) and thus enter the vascular system directly. They then reach other organs through the blood stream where they can settle and multiply. These metastases are frequently far removed from the primary tumour. In these cases we talk of remote metastases.

When tumours have invaded the lymphatic system or the veins, it is likely that the primary tumour spreads via the lymph and blood vessels and develops metastases.

At the time of its removal the primary tumour has often already developed tiny micrometastases which can present as remote metastases at a later stage. The removal of a primary tumour therefore doesn't necessarily complete the healing process. We have to do everything in our power to prevent possible micrometastases from further developing.

If metastases don't possess the network of blood vessels that feeds them, they can't degenerate into dangerous tumours. In this context a substance called *angiostatin* has been proven to play a significant part in the regeneration of blood vessels.

Angiostatin – Enemy of the metastases

Angiostatin is a protein that inhibits angioneogenesis (the regeneration of blood vessels). The American physician Judah Folkman has established that large primary tumours produce angiostatin which prevents the growth of metastases by blocking the regeneration of blood vessels, thereby cutting off the metastases' nutrient supply.

One could say that the primary tumour doesn't want to lose its dominance over the metastases and keeps them under control (see Figure 11). Through angiostatin the metastases remain in a dormant state without, however, losing their malign potential.

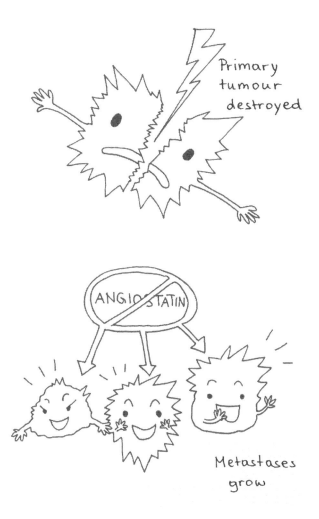

Primary
tumour
destroyed

ANGIOSTATIN

Metastases
grow

Fig. 11: When the primary tumour is removed (through
surgery or radiotherapy for instance), it is possible that
small micro-metastases present in the body are no longer
held in check through the primary tumour's angiostatin.
The danger of the metastases' accelerated growth increases.

How to counteract metastatic spread after the removal of the primary tumour

Some drugs can counteract the formation and growth of metastases. They do, however, cause a number of side effects so that prolonged use can be problematic.

But there are foods and food supplements that have a similar antiangiogenic effect on cancer cells to that of angiostatin. They include:

- *Foodstuffs:* linseed, garlic, ginseng, green tea, pomegranate, tomatoes, turmeric, cabbage, parsley, chives and many more
- *Food supplements:* Curcumin, green tea extract, pomegranate concentrate, MSM, salvestrols, milk thistle and many more

As inflammations directly trigger the growth of new blood vessels, it can generally be said that everything leading to a reduction of inflammations also counteracts cancer.

Anything boosting our body's immune system also supplies us with more strength in our fight against malignant tumours and metastases.

My diet change begins

When we have a strong immune system, our white blood cells are also very active. These include *natural killer cells* (abbreviated to *NK cells*) which can obstruct the formation of tumours and metastases. NK cells, as their name implies, can kill tumour cells. Once they recognise a cancer cell they "shoot" their ammunition (perforin) at it and e enzymes (granzymes) through its damaged membrane, thereby prompting the cancer cell's apoptosis.

Recognition of cancer cells can be facilitated by taking enzymes. Because chronic inflammations promote the cancer's spreading, any anti-inflammatory measures, especially anti-inflammatory foods, counteract cancer. The lower the inflammatory markers – they can be measured by blood tests – the longer the patient is likely to live. If the tumour's nutrient supply through the blood vessels is also successfully withdrawn, the patient has practically won. As already mentioned, some foodstuffs counteract the regeneration of blood vessels (angioneogenesis) and as such possess anticarcinogenic properties.

Knowing this, I started to change my diet and also took the first food supplements. In April 2011 I began taking Echinacea, as well as an enzyme preparation and selenium. Milk thistle to support the detoxification of my liver completed my nutritional supplement programme for the time being.

The first small successes

Armed with these dietary supplements, I accompanied my family on a two week holiday at the seaside. The days consisted long barefoot walks on the beach in the morning to "ground" myself, and in the clean sea to supply my skin and respiratory system with salt, magnesium, iodine and other important trace elements. Maritime aerosols, minute saline water droplets inhaled through the moist sea air, are especially beneficial for our health. Fresh Mediterranean food with plenty of vegetables, regional small fish and fresh fruit made the holidays complete. To my delight the dream of my facial nerves' recovery started to become a little bit of a reality after those two weeks. Pretty much six months to the day after the radiotherapy I suddenly noticed that I occasionally managed very slight facial movements of the right side of my face although it took enormous effort. From then on my facial nerves began to regenerate noticeably, if extremely slowly.

My grandmother has always been convinced that "sand, salt, sun and sea" are good for your health. Now I follow her advice and spend at least three weeks by the sea every year since my cancer was diagnosed. Always at a time when it's hot enough to go swimming and I can take full advantage of nature's "all inclusive package deal".

Scary first check-up

For my first follow-up in August 2011 I had been recommended a clinic with a high resolution MRI scanner.

Viewing the images it was very obvious for me that my tumour had been substantially destroyed and only a thickened nerve remained. I felt extremely relieved seeing that tumours rarely ever break down. But the specialist put a damper on my initial joy when he told us that the nerve shouldn't look like that. My mother was speechless. Yet I still felt that the images couldn't have been better. During the course of our conversation it became apparent that the doctor had assessed the images based on the presumption that I'd had previous surgery, when he repeatedly pointed out that the area in question shouldn't appear the way it did. The problem therefore was not my thickened nerve but that the doctor simply wasn't used to evaluating post carbon ion therapy MRI scans. So I remained completely calm while my mother was a nervous wreck for a while. Not until the afternoon did I finally convince her that we actually had reason to rejoice.

This example quite clearly illustrates the importance of prior research into the most up-to-date radiotherapies depending on the area of application, side effects and aftercare. This was an important factor, amongst others, which motivated me to write this book.

I now have my MRI scans done at a radiology institute with excellent imaging equipment. The results are always reliably evaluated by the same physician. A physician who knows me and my medical history more than well enough to properly assess the scans. This should turn out to be extremely helpful later on.

Inspired by the extensive destruction of my tumour and the beginning of my nerve regeneration, I started to broaden my research into nutrition and dietary supplements to keep supporting my body's healing process as much as possible.

The importance of a proper diet and dietary supplements

After months of research I gradually started to understand that there are many factors which can help the body to protect itself from cancer if properly applied.

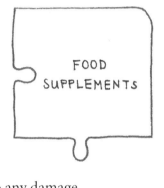

FOOD SUPPLEMENTS

Today I realise that our body hosts millions of precursor cancer cells. A healthy immune system easily keeps these cells in check and wards them off so they can't do any damage.

To what extent cancer can be influenced by our lifestyle and diet becomes particularly apparent when we realise that the disease differs immensely in its worldwide prevalence and types. Many kinds of cancer, like prostate, breast and bowel cancer, for example, are far more common in the western hemisphere than in Asia.

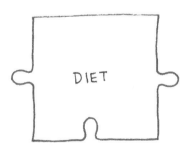

DIET

According to estimates, 30 percent of all cancers are connected to individual eating habits. Studies established a close relationship between insufficient fruit and vegetable consumption and the increase of some cancer types. Certain foods facilitate tumours, whilst others stunt their growth so that they can exist as undiagnosed, harmless microtumours for an entire lifespan.

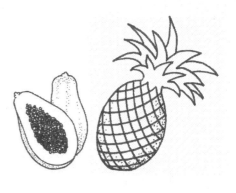

At my first meeting with some people suffering from the same disease, I was told that our kind of cancer is caused by a congenital genetic defect and therefore not susceptible to treatment. But I am convinced that the adenoid cystic carcinoma (ACC) is a genetic defect acquired during one's lifetime.

If my type of cancer had been attributable to a congenital genetic defect it would hardly explain why it occurs at the age of 18 in some people and at 70 in others. Those different times of onset could only be explained by immune systems of varying strength. Not all those with a congenital predisposition suffer from cancer.

I believe that the immune system is always responsible for our wellbeing and everyone can influence this to a certain extent.

Before starting to take food supplements, it is advisable to have a blood test to determine the actual status. I therefore regularly (once or twice a year) have an extensive immune status test and insist on including Immunophenotyping, a lymphocyte function analysis, inflammation and rheumatism serology (CRP), vitamin D and selenium levels in addition to the differential blood count. Our immune system contains helper cells which assist in activating its NK cells. The NK cells then locate mutated cells and destroy them. But the immune system also contains suppressor cells which can deactivate the NK cells. Because cancer cells don't want to be attacked, they generate more suppressor cells and activate them. For that reason an extensive immune status test doesn't only measure NK cells but also helper and suppressor cells.

As the lymphocyte subpopulations also reflect feelings of helplessness and other psychological states, patients who are better equipped to psychologically deal with a disease have more active NK cells than those who give up and succumb to helplessness and depression. The more active the NK cells, the higher the patient's chances of survival.

→ **My Advice:** Ensure that all results are immediately handed or posted to you. It's extremely tedious having to chase after them although they are urgently needed for further consultations. Unfortunately I have quite often heard of clinics or doctors not being willing to release the results for weeks. On the day of the check-up I therefore insisted that I would take the images with me immediately and that I would like the results to be sent to me. If necessary I'll also wait for a few hours at the hospital and pay a small contribution towards the costs.

After the examination I always have the doctor explain all results in detail and when it comes to my blood values I'm never happy whenever they are in the lower reference range.

Vitamin D and selenium levels play a major part in cancer prevention, treatment and aftercare. Both levels should always be close to the upper limit of the reference range. Especially selenium levels are closely linked to one's diet and can vary enormously. It is therefore important to keep having them checked to ensure proper nutrition.

Food supplements during chemo-, immuno- or radiotherapy

When taking food supplements during chemo-, immuno- or radiotherapy one has to bear in mind that food supplements can influence these conventional treatments.

The success of orthodox oncological treatments partly depends on the desired production of oxygen free radicals to attack the tumour cells and initiate deadly response mechanisms. Food supplements with antioxidant properties which destroy oxygen radicals can diminish the effect of conventional treatment when taken parallel to it.

The use of food supplements during treatment should therefore definitely be discussed with the attending physician.

Selenium, however, seems to be an exception. Numerous studies confirm that selenium apparently not only has an anti-cancer effect but also protects healthy cells from damages through conventional cancer treatments such as radio- or chemotherapies. Selenium is even said to render chemotherapy more effective. If administered in time it can prevent resistance to cytostatics or resensitise tumour cells to the effect of chemotherapeutic agents.

Trials also showed that *sulforaphane* can increase the effect of conventional cancer medication (Sorafenib) and possibly make tumour stem cells more vulnerable towards chemotherapy. Ingrid Herr, the head of the Surgical Research Dept. at the University Clinic in Heidelberg, could prove that the effect of *Sorafenib*, a drug frequently used against cancer in conventional medicine, can be improved when taken in combination with sulforaphane. Furthermore, sulforaphane can protect healthy cells from possible DNA damages through Sorafenib. Taking sulforaphane during chemotherapy can therefore enhance its success. In its concentrated form sulforaphane is found in broccoli sprouts.

Milk thistle compounds can counteract the frequent nausea associated with chemotherapy or possible liver damage caused by the administration of cytostatics. It is a liver restorative, detoxifying and considered to be the most important plant to protect the liver.

Last but not least, I should mention that a high *vitamin D level* as well as a sufficient intake of *OMEGA 3 fatty acids* promotes health. For cancer patients it is therefore advisable to provide the body adequately with both during treatment. It is also very important to always *drink plenty of fluids* during chemo-, radio- or immunotherapy, provided one's body allows it. Water and unsweetened herbal teas support the body during toxin egestion!

Why don't more medical practitioners recommend a change of diet?

I have developed the lovely tradition of chatting to my personal physicians over a nice dinner once a year. During one of these evenings I told the physicians about my general health and the supplements and foodstuffs I take to prevent the cancer from recurring. They were very pleased about my wellbeing and also interested in my preventative supplemental diet, however they were also sceptical. They believed the area had not yet been sufficiently researched.

Of course, anticarcinogenic foods will never be as intensively researched as pharmaceuticals which generate billions in revenue. Most of all, they won't be advertised to the general public because natural anticarcinogenic foods cannot be patented or considerable amounts of money be made from them. In addition, a change in diet often doesn't produce positive results as fast as medication does. As such physicians are used to and trained to prescribe drugs, not to recommend foods.

However, the extremely varied worldwide cancer rates are extremely impressive and show definite connections between diet and cancer. As natural foodstuffs generally don't have any harmful side effects, cancer patients as well as healthy people can only benefit from their conscious, selective intake as a preventative. Especially those who have or had cancer shouldn't leave any stones unturned. At one stage I doubted if the health food constituents could actually reach all my cells. I was standing in a garden looking at a gigantic tree and thought: "This large tree feeds all its leaves, up to its very top, through its roots!"

Then I understood that everything we eat affects our entire body. But we have to take into account that the brain-blood barrier, which protects the brain from pathogens circulating in the blood, can also prevent potential active substances from reaching the brain. Food supplements able to surmount the brain-blood barrier and which are also supposed to affect brain tumour cells include curcumin, for example.

What to consider
in anti-cancer diets

There are countless books and even more opinions regarding the proper diet during and after cancer. Having read extensively about the subject and also tested many of the suggestions, I would like to explain selected approaches I personally consider to be important in more detail.

An alkaline environment

In the short term most natural healing methods are based on a complete alkaline diet with an interruption of the supply of acid-forming foods. The term "alkaline" doesn't mean that the foodstuff has an alkaline pH value, but that it delivers alkaline minerals to the organism or triggers endogenous alkaline activation. We are therefore concerned with how food affects the body and what substances develop during metabolisation. In the long term a healthy diet should contain excess alkalines, i.e. consist of 70 to 80 percent alkaline-forming foods and the rest of healthy acid-forming foods.

My wake-up call was the discovery that an over-acidic body tries to neutralise its organism itself. The pH value of the blood to facilitate our body's optimal functioning lies at 7.4 and should only minimally fluctuate. To maintain a value of 7.4, the organism has to constantly provide alkaline substances. Here calcium plays a significant part. When the alkaline buffers in the body are depleted through an over-acidic diet, the body uses calcium from the bones for acid buffering. To maintain healthy bones a mostly alkaline diet with plenty of fruit and vegetables is unavoidable.

Alkaline foods which also contain valuable calcium include: green leafy vegetables (such as collard greens, rocket and dandelion) as well as linseed, lentils, white beans, sesame seeds and soya beans. Magnesium is also an alkaline mineral and should be adequately included in the diet. Pulses, bananas and nettles, for instance, are high in magnesium.

Quinoa, tasty and priced by the Incas, is a particularly valuable grain with regard to minerals as it contains large amounts of potassium, magnesium and iron.

Taking potassium and magnesium, or even better potassium- and magnesium citrate (citrates are these minerals' organic compounds and increase their bioavailability), additionally improves bone health. This happens because the potassium citrate contributes towards calcium remaining in the bones and not getting into the blood. A study has proven that high amounts of calcium in the blood more than double the death risk in the case of aggressive, poorly differentiated prostate carcinomas.

Taken together with silicon, vitamin D, vitamin K (see later chapters) and lots of exercise our bones will stay strong well into old age.

To establish if you are following the correct diet and your acid-base balance is okay, you can easily measure the pH by dipping a test strip into a urine sample. The urine's

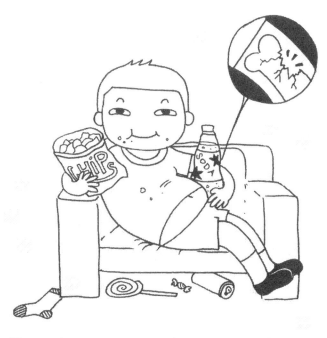

Fig. 12: An inactive person has an over-acidic system through the consumption of meat, cheese, sweets, white bread, biscuits, soft drinks etc. The calcium in the bones is used up, resulting in porous (brittle) bones.

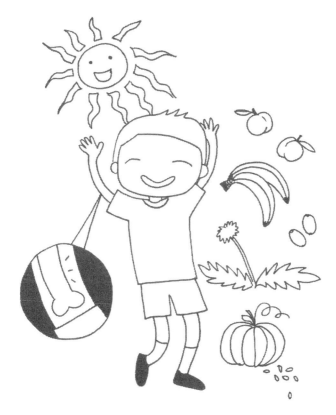

*Fig. 13: An active person has an alkaline system through
a vegetarian diet consisting of green leafy vegetables,
pulses, cabbage etc. Calcium is provided by the food,
resulting in healthy bones.*

pH describes its acidity which particularly depends on your diet. The results should fluctuate because this means that the body naturally regulates the acid-base balance. The pH should be at its lowest in the morning. During my radiotherapy I measured my pH several times a day and ensured that all values after 10 am showed a pH of roughly 6.5 or more.

Since having been diagnosed with cancer, I generally try to eat as much alkaline-generating foods as possible. In the morning I ideally chew some fresh herbs like basil or thyme or, if I can make myself, drink a glass of sauerkraut juice before having coffee. To prepare me for a healthy start to the day, I let two Japanese umeboshi (Japanese fruit, a kind of apricot, preserved in salt, also called the "queen of alkaline foods") slowly melt on my tongue. Even today, nearly seven years after my radiotherapy, I try to follow this routine as far as I can.

Sugar alert!

There are multiple types of sugar but not all of them have a sweet taste. Single, double and certain multiple sugars (maltodextrin and maltotriose) are also called mono-, di-, and oligosaccharides and have a sweet taste. Multiple sugars called polysaccharides (starch and cellulose) however, are neutral in taste. Monosaccharides are the basic building blocks of carbohydrates. Before the human body can use saccharides (carbohydrates), they have to be broken down into their monosaccharides in the small intestine. But carbohydrates differ in their effect on blood sugar levels. Only carbohydrates, which slowly make the blood sugar levels rise, should be recommended i.e. have a low glycaemic index (GI). This index measures the ability of foodstuffs to increase blood sugar levels compared to the effect of glucose.

Foods which only slowly cause blood sugar levels to rise include:

- vegetables like courgettes, broccoli, red cabbage or lentils and
- fruit like oranges, apples or pears.

Brown rice, oat flakes, wholemeal bread and sweet potatoes also have a relatively low glycaemic index. For a healthy diet

110

it is generally important to ensure keeping blood sugar levels as constant as possible.

Foodstuffs with large amounts of household sugars (sucrose), glucose or malt sugar (maltose) should be avoided because they quickly cause blood sugar levels to rise. The body reacts by secreting insulin.

In turn, insulin, a hormone produced in the pancreas, facilitates the quick absorption of the single sugar glucose (a type of the digested sugar in the body) from the blood into the cells. So-called insulin peaks, a sudden rapid rise of insulin levels, enable the cancer cells to grow and more easily penetrate the surrounding tissue because insulin is generally a growth factor.

Those wanting to prevent cancer should severely limit their intake of quickly digestible carbohydrates such as glucose/ dextrose, chips, cornflakes, white bread and soft drinks. The aim is to combine foodstuffs in a way to reduce insulin peaks. This works with foods which only make the insulin level rise slowly, i.e. foods with a low glycaemic Index. Wine should be enjoyed with the meal and not on its own. Sweets, if one can't do without, should be eaten as a dessert and not in between.

The fact that cancer cells greedily love glucose is exploited by the imaging technique *FDG-PET* (short for fluorodeoxyglucose positron emission tomography) in the diagnosis of tumours. The patient is injected with a radioactive glucose solution which is absorbed by the cancer cells and enhances their visibility.

The fact that cancer cells love sugar could, in my view, also be exploited in the treatment of some cases of cancer. Sugar could act like a Trojan horse that causes the cancer cells to open their "mouths" wide.

If honey or maple syrup, for instance, is mixed with anti-carcinogenic substances, the cancer cell can be tricked into absorbing them. When fancying something sweet, this can be taken as a combination of honey, curcumin, linseed oil

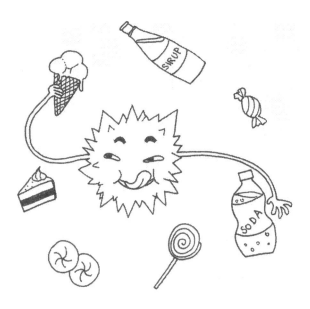

Fig. 14: Cancer cells love sugar and multiply – malignant tumours grow.

and black pepper blended into a paste. Apart from using sugar as a Trojan horse, however, one should limit its intake as much as possible.

The scientist Johannes F. Coy explains the danger of food-stuffs containing sugar. Through its *fast glucose release (insulin peaks) sugar provides the basis for the tumour cells switching from combustion* (oxygen-dependent energy release) *to fermentation* (non-oxygen-dependent energy release with formation of lactic acid).

Coy believes that tumours are principally benign at first. These benign tumour cells divide and merely push healthy neighbouring cells aside, but don't destroy them. Their growth behaviour is therefore non-invasive. At this stage the cells have not as yet mutated into malignant cancer cells.

Only once tumour cells switch from combustion to fermentation do they become malignant, he maintains.

How to prevent tumour cells from switching to anaerobic digestion

According to Coy it is important to avoid insulin peaks and to primarily eat foods with a low *glycaemic index* to prevent possibly present tumour cells from switching to anaerobic digestion. The lower the body sugar level is, the more uncomfortable the cancer cell feels.

Tumour growth can be compared to the rabbit plague in Australia. The rabbits had been introduced from Europe and conditions for them to multiply were (and are) ideal. They had lots of food and had almost hardly any natural predators. So not just the rabbits but also the excellent conditions are responsible for their rapid breeding.

Something similar applies to cancer cells. If they are well nourished and their enemies are too weak and/or cannot recognise their malignant intent, they multiply inexorably.

A typical western diet, rich in sugar and processed foods, increases the risk of falling ill many times over as compared to a typical Asian diet, for example. Sugar generally causes chronic inflammations in the body and chronic inflammations in turn facilitate diseases like diabetes or cancer.

The by now huge sugar consumption is on average close to 83 pounds per person in the European Union in 2014/2015. It had its origin in the middle of the 19th century, the end of common self-sufficiency and the start of mass-produced foods rich in sugar and starch.

I try to severely reduce my intake of carbohydrates that lead to peaks in blood sugar and insulin levels. For that reason white bread, pasta, baked goods and sweets hardly feature at all in my diet!

Critical evaluation of foodstuffs really brought it home to me how much sugar I can avoid every day: no sugar in tea or coffee, no white bread, no extra sugar in yoghurts or fruit juices (the homemade variety tastes better anyway) no soft drinks (cola, lemonade, iced tea, energy drinks) and no convenience foods. If it really has to be something sweet, it should be combined with healthy foods like fruit and vegetables. This reduces cancer-conducive insulin peaks. For my smoothies, if a banana isn't already sweet enough, I use raisins or liquorice root to sweeten it and it tastes wonderful. Agave nectar or syrup is another suitable sweetener. I allow myself chocolate from 70 percent cocoa content upwards, any organic fruit and whole-grain products.

→ **My Advice:** Cancer patients have often clearly lost weight even before their diagnosis. But as they need sufficient strength to fight the disease, sugar reduction should be a gradual process to avoid hypoglycaemia (low blood sugar). After a few weeks of slowly reducing sugar and the associated dietary changes, however, they will more than likely feel significantly better.

My recipe for protein bread with almonds:
Ingredients: 4 whole eggs, 320 g lean curd, 200 g ground almonds, 2 level tsp baking powder, 2 tbs soya flower, bread seasoning, salt, ground coriander, ground fenugreek, walnuts, sunflower seeds, pumpkin seeds or linseed according to taste.
Preparation: Whip the eggs until foamy, then stir in the curd and the rest of the ingredients.

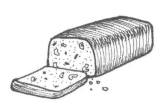

Line a loaf pan with baking paper and bake for roughly 50 minutes at 180 °C. Should the dough cling to a toothpick when pricked with it, reduce the temperature to 150 °C.

Coconut oil

Coconut oil consists mainly of medium-chain fatty acids which the body can resorb without the aid of digestive enzymes and bile acid. It is therefore ideal for people with digestive disorders. Coconut oil minimally deposits in the adipose tissue (fatty tissue). Instead the body prefers using it for energy 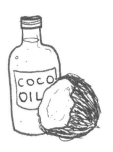 production. The medium-chain fatty acids are changed into ketones in the liver and used as a fuel source by most body cells. Ketones barely influence blood sugar levels and larger insulin peaks – as is the case with glucose – don't occur.

As already mentioned, cancer cells feed on sugar and have on average ten times as many insulin receptors on their surface than normal cells. Cancer cells may possibly die when trying to starve them by depriving the body of any type of sugar. But the patient may die even faster, unless this is counteracted. Fats and their building blocks can remedy this to a certain extent. Tumour cells practically don't utilise fatty acids at all. Coconut oil, for instance, can provide healthy cells with fuel (ketones) without nourishing the cancer cells because these have no use for it. Especially the lauric acid in coconut oil fights bacteria and viruses. The caprylic acid contained in coconut oil is an effective remedy for fungal infections.

Coconut water and coconuts are also very healthy and rich in vitamins, minerals and amino acids. Personally, I use coconut oil and desiccated coconut (selenium) every day in my smoothies and add a teaspoon of coconut oil and a little cinnamon to my coffee. In addition I use coconut oil on my hair and skin and even treat burns with it. I like drinking coconut water and feel that it benefits my joints. This may be attributable to its high mineral content of chlorine, potassium, magnesium, sodium, phosphor and sulphur.

Coconut oil and coconut fat can be heated to around 200 °C (during frying) with little risk of developing carcinogenic substances, in comparison with other major cooking oils. It is therefore advisable to use only oils with a high smoke point when frying. The smoke point is the temperature where the oil shows a clearly visible bluish smoke when heated. I try to avoid this stage in the first place.

Smoothies

Smoothies are mostly made from whole pureed fruit or vegetables including skin, seeds and pips. I've bought myself a special smoothie maker and enjoy preparing the delicious drink nearly every day.

Fresh fruit and vegetable juices are a wonderful way to provide the body with large amounts of anti-cancer agents. Juices should be drunk right after their preparation as soon after chemical reactions set in which can alter and devalue its substances. Antioxidants, for instance, have not yet oxidised and can therefore intercept oxygen radicals in the body and render them harmless. Like good wine, vegetable juices should linger on the palate for a while so their active agents can also be absorbed through the oral mucosa. Fruit juices, however, should be swallowed straight away so their acids don't attack dental enamel.

Two smoothie recipes for inspiration:

Rich fruit smoothie:
Ingredients: 1 pomegranate (contains valuable ellagic acid; remove the red outer skin), ½ organic lemon (with skin and seeds – Vitamin C), 1 mango or a piece of papaya (papaya contains the important enzyme papain; use only a

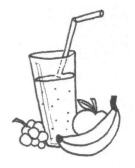

few (!) of the seeds or the smoothie will taste too peppery), 1 apple (whole with pips but without stalk), 1 banana (peeled), 1 tbs desiccated coconut (selenium), 1 tsp coconut oil or linseed oil, 1 tbs oat flakes (silicon), linseed, browntop millet, psyllium husks (for a more viscous consistency if desired), 1 tsp/tablet curcumin (powder) (careful: curcumin leaves lasting yellow stains!), water, raisins or liquorice root powder (to sweeten).

Refreshing green smoothie:
Ingredients: 1 apple (whole with pips but without stalk) 1 banana (peeled), ½ organic lemon (with skin and seeds), nettles, moringa or papaya leaves, fresh mint, oats, ground tigernuts, a few briefly soaked chia seeds, 1 tsp flower pollen, water.

Mix all the ingredients together and blend well.

Balance between free radicals and antioxidants

Apart from a permanently high sugar consumption in connection with insulin peaks and a constantly acidotic environment in the body, developing cancer is also facilitated by a prevalence of free radicals. But what are they actually? How do they develop and how do they work?

Free radicals

Free radicals are positively charged, tiny atoms or molecules with one or several unpaired electrons.

They continuously form in our body through natural metabolic processes. The most important of these is the oxygen radical. It plays a vital role in the fight against foreign organisms. In the case of bacterial inflammations the defence cells develop aggressive oxygen radicals which can help them to destroy aggressive pathogens. As such free radicals are not exclusively bad but even possess an important function. If an immune system is too weak, however, the development of free radicals gets out of hand and they no longer just fight aggressive pathogens but also start damaging the organism.

But they don't want to remain "single" and therefore steal an electron from stable pairs (stable molecules), like someone who interferes in a relationship and steals someone else's partner. The one who's left behind now also becomes a free radical in search of a partnership. At all costs, the newly single free radical will abduct a partner (electron) from a stable partnership in order to regain stability. This leads to a never ending chain reaction where "singles" (free radicals – positively charged molecules or atoms) steal an electron

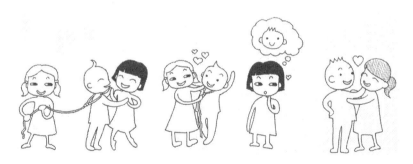

Fig. 15: Oxidation: a free radical steels an electron from stable pairs (stable molecules) to enter into a stable partnership itself. A new free radical is created which now also looks for a partner. A chain reaction ensues.

from other pairs (stable molecules) and thus create new free radicals (singles) (see Figure 15).

This chemical reaction is called *oxidation* and always follows the same pattern: One substance (=electron acceptor) takes one or more electrons from another substance (= electron donor).

A similar process occurs when iron starts to rust. Here an oxygen molecule (electron acceptor) steals an electron from an iron molecule (electron donor) and rust appears. Another example is an apple with a bite taken out and left – it oxidises and turns brown.

Once the free radicals (parts of the oxygen molecules) come in contact with body cells they also steel an electron from the cell molecules.

Such chain reactions can alter vital molecules in the body through wrong pairings in their structures, particularly in their genetic material. Should these molecular changes affect the DNA, the resulting defects can contribute towards causing cancer. An excess of free radicals in the blood can be verified by monitoring the oxidation state through measuring the redox potential. In the case of too many free radicals in the blood we talk of increased oxidative stress. Counteracting this with natural vitamins, enzymes, trace elements and secondary plant compounds is particularly important.

By now free radicals are associated with the development of more than 50 diseases, one of them cancer. They are certainly never the sole catalyst, but play their part as an "accomplice".

The development of free radicals is facilitated by:
- smoke (exhaust fumes, cigarettes and cigars)
- UV light
- increased stress hormones
- electromagnetic rays (mobile phones, WLAN, TVs, computers)
- unhealthy diet

- pollutants in the household and environment such as preservatives and chemicals
- drugs
- medication: antibiotics, cytostatics.

As electromagnetic rays also facilitate the development of free radicals and thereby contribute towards causing cancer, I recommend being careful when using mobile phones, WLAN etc. The radiation is even further increased by metals in or on the body such as dental braces, metal fasteners, zips, key-rings and others which can attract the radiation like an antenna. When I wore braces I could literally feel the radiation when my face turned red and puffy following a short chat on my mobile phone. Now I make sure that any new phone I buy has a low SAR value. I also activate the speaker and hold the mobile as far away from my body as possible. Besides, I avoid carrying it in my pockets and close to zips and store it in my handbag or backpack. I also make sure that my bras have no metal wires and aren't too tight so they don't exert pressure on the lymphatic system. The lymphatic and circulatory system is in particular responsible for transporting oxygen and nutrients to the cells and removing metabolic residue and toxins. Cancer development can be promoted if this process is interrupted.

Smokers should be aware that the body suffers from chronic inflammations caused by its continuous fight against toxins. This infection defence also causes the formation of free oxygen radicals. It is therefore hardly surprising that roughly 30 percent of all cancer deaths are attributable to smoking. Once smokers stop the habit, the originally increased energy demand to fight chronic inflammations decreased, frequently accompanied by weight gain. Quite contrary to cancer patients who often lose weight because tumour cells need large amounts of energy and also rob other cells of their nutrition. If the cause of weight loss is unknown, one should therefore have it investigated.

As cancer can be favoured by many harmful influences, it is important to counteract them through a healthy diet with plenty of antioxidants to create a balance.

So I took at closer look at antioxidants which protect our body cells from harmful free radicals.

Antioxidants – Counteracting free radicals

Antioxidants are complex chemical compounds which can prevent or delay oxidation. They occur naturally in the organisms of mammals or plants, but today they can also be synthetically produced. In the human body they counteract free radicals.

Plants have also developed antioxidants to protect themselves. As they are to a large extent exposed to the same environmental influences as humans, their antioxidants can also help humans to stay healthy.

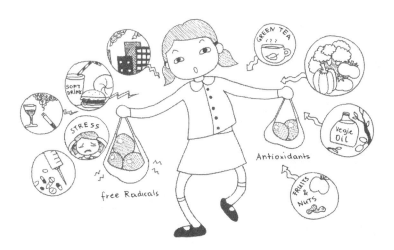

Fig. 16: Imbalance between free radicals and antioxidants.

Antioxidants include:

- *trace elements* like *selenium* (in coconuts, Brazil nuts), *zinc* (in crustaceans like oysters and in whole grain oats, pumpkin seeds, linseed, poppy seeds, millet, amaranth)
- *vitamin E* (in plant-based oils like wheat germ oil, olive oil, sunflower oil, safflower oil, nuts and wholemeal products)
  Vitamin E can interrupt the free radicals' chain reaction because it can release an electron without changing into a reactive, aggressive molecule itself.
  Warning: Recent studies showed overdosing can occur, especially if high doses of vitamin E are taken as a food supplement.
- *secondary plant compounds* such as flavonoids (in green tea, dried herbs, dandelions), polyphenols (in apples, berries, pomegranates), lycopene (especially in cooked tomatoes) and sulforaphane (in broccoli)
- *enzymes* like *coenzyme Q10* (in beef, chicken, fish, soya oils and nuts)
- *vitamin C* (e.g. in acerola cherries, fresh rosehips, green peppers, kale, white cabbage, lemons, sweet potatoes, chives, kohlrabi)
  A vitamin C deficiency can be recognized by reduced performance capacity and susceptibility to infections.
- *astaxanthin*, a carotenoid with antioxidant effect
- *vitamin A*, only occurs in animal products, especially liver products
  Vegetables contain a vitamin A precursor called beta-carotene. The body can convert it into a usable form of vitamin A. Carrots, kale, spinach and pumpkins, for example, have a high proportion of beta-carotene.
- *turmeric* and *curcumin*

Turmeric and Curcumin

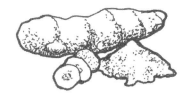

Turmeric, also called yellow ginger, a plant that can grow up to 40 inches, is originally from South Asia. Turmeric powder can be ground from its dried rootstock/rhizome. In the food industry turmeric is used as a dye also known as E100.

Seven years ago, when I found out about the effect of Curcumin, an extract from Turmeric (lat. Curcuma Longa), it hadn't been quite as extensively studied as today. A quick research only revealed a single experiment with mice whose cancer had been successfully combated with a curcumin infusion.

Nowadays numerous studies exist about curcumin's medicinal properties. A contributing factor may be that since 2009, Curcumin the turmeric plant's main active ingredient, can be extracted in a more advanced and efficient way through ultrasound. Curcumin has been proven to be effective in a multitude of complaints and diseases. It's been used in traditional Chinese and Ayurvedic medicine for centuries if not millennia.

In my opinion, Curcumin is the best anti-cancer agent of all, as its effect has now been substantiated in numerous studies of nearly all cancer types.

In 2005 turmeric was recognised as the only natural remedy in the prevention and treatment of cancer at a medical conference in the United States, regardless of the cancer type. Curcumin can easily break down the blood-brain barrier.

In India, breast, prostate, lung and colon cancer occur on average nine times less frequently than in the USA. This is attributed to the high consumption of turmeric and thus a high dose of curcumin in the Indian diet.

Curcumin works on practically all our billions of body cells and protects them from attacks by "single" aggressive free radicals. Not having this protection can lead to functional impairments and cell mutations which can ultimately cause countless complaints including cancer.

As already mentioned, the best way to protect ourselves from free radicals is to take so-called antioxidants such as curcumin.

Turmeric or more specifically Curcumin is particularly interesting as it wages war against cancer on several levels:

1. Curcumin inhibits the lactic acid creating glyoxalase 1 enzyme in cancer cells which produces laevorotatory lactic acid. Thus the cancer cells produce less lactic acid and are more easily assailable by the immune system.

2. Curcumin stimulates the immune system and increases the white blood cells' activity.

3. Curcumin also increases the protective p53 tumour suppressor's activity and can therefore prevent cells from mutating. When a healthy cell is going to divide, activating p53 is usually unnecessary (see Figure 17a). When a DNA-damaged cell divides, activating p53 repairs the damaged cell before division or drives it to it's programmed cell-death (Figure 17b). This can stop the growth and spread of tumours and impair the formation of metastases. If p53 is not activated in a damaged cell, mutation defects can occur during cell division (Figure 17c).

4. Curcumin prevents the development of blood vessels in the tumour tissue, thus impairing the tumour's supply and arresting cancer cell division.

5. Storing curcumin in cancer cells' membranes renders them more unstable and as such more assailable by the immune system's helper cells.

6. Curcumin has the ability to defeat NF-kappa B (the inflammatory response released by tumour cells).

7. Curcumin can bypass the blood-brain barrier and therefore also positively affect brain tumours.

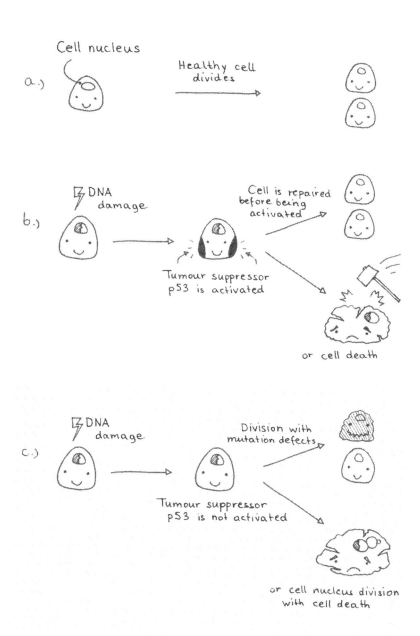

Fig. 17: Cell division with mutation defects.

8. As a strong antioxidant curcumin provides protection from free radicals.
9. Curcumin fights inflammations by lowering histamine levels.
10. Curcumin promotes more stable blood sugar levels. It should therefore be taken with your meals.
11. Curcumin can deactivate the Galectin 3 protein which plays a part in the spreading of cancer and the formation of metastases. A highly significant connection between increased Galectin 3 values and shorter survival rates has also been found in patients presenting with the same disease as mine (ACC). So curcumin can lower Galectin 3 levels and therefore influence the expected life expectancy extremely positively.

Beside its promising effect on cancer, curcumin also works for many other diseases and complaints. I would like to list some of these here as I have personally witnessed curcumin's positive effect on friends and acquaintances:

1. Intestinal polyps - regression and non-recurrence
2. Arthrosis/arthritis – taking curcumin significantly relieves the pain
3. Allergies
4. Acts against herpes viruses and accelerates healing
5. Rashes
6. Itching
7. Flatulence
8. Regulates digestion
9. Possibly combats arteriosclerosis and vascular deposits as well as having a slight blood-thinning effect which can also lower the risk of strokes and heart attacks
10. Detoxifies and regulates blood pressure

I recommend taking at least three times 1000 mg of curcumin daily in tablet form with black pepper for prevention and aftercare. Ensure not to exceed the proportion of 5 mg of pepper per 1000 mg tablet.

The combination of curcumin (or turmeric respectively) and pepper is important as this makes it easier to pass through the intestinal barrier. The organism's absorption is aided by the piperine contained in pepper which can massively increase the effect (up to 2000 times). Adding a small spoon of high-quality oil is meant to increase the body's absorption of curcumin even more and ease breaking through the blood-brain barrier.

Therefore when cooking I frequently use turmeric with black pepper and oil. It is important to lightly sauté the turmeric in heatable oil because this increases its effect. Now and then I drink a cup of warm milk (soya, rice or lactose-free cow milk) with a teaspoon of turmeric (here it is important to exclusively use Bio turmeric powder from the healthfood shop) and sweetened with a little honey in the evening. In the morning turmeric or curcumin can be mixed into a muesli or smoothie.

Be careful in case of gallbladder problems as curcumin stimulates the gallbladder and can possibly overstrain it. If, however, the gallbladder has been removed, curcumin is generally well tolerated, but stomach pains can occur when the intestines or the digestion no longer function properly or are already too badly damaged. In this case curcumin intake should definitely be reduced to an extent where the pain subsides. I don't advise taking anything with antiangiogenetic properties, i.e. preventing vascularisation, during pregnancy as this could interfere with the embryo's development.

Taking vitamin D is supposed to further heighten curcumin's effect. Curcumin on its own already causes a measurable increase of the protein cathelicidin, an organic compound of several amino acids which fight bacteria in the immune system. The protein's value, enhanced by curcumin, increases even more in the body if vitamin D is taken in addition. This enables the immune system to fight pathogens and inflammations more successfully.

Selenium and vitamin D

Extensive studies have shown that the probability of cancer recurrence is significantly higher in people with low selenium and vitamin D levels. So I had my selenium and vitamin D blood levels measured. Unfortunately both values were low.

Selenium

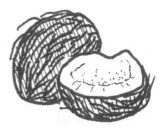

Selenium is a vital trace element which has to be absorbed through our diet.

It is so important for the human body because it is incorporated into molecules of the so-called glutathione peroxidase (GPx) enzyme family. The GPx enzyme develops its maximum activity at a selenium concentration in whole blood from 140 to 160 µg/l. Selenium enables the enzyme to ensure the faultless functioning of all cell membranes to combat oxidative stress.

Research has shown that countries where the soil is low in selenium have significantly higher cancer rates than those with selenium-rich soil.

With the help of selenium, harmful cytotoxins are quickly eliminated and premature cell attrition prevented. This also provides the basis for using selenium in cancer treatment. It assists regular cell division and can therefore arrest the division and further development of tumour cells. It also reduces serious side effects caused by medication. Good results have so far been achieved in the treatment of lung, prostate, breast, colon and liver cancer.

> *The effect of conventional treatments such as chemo- or radiotherapy is also enhanced by taking selenium because it makes the cancer cells more vulnerable while simultaneously protecting healthy cells. During radiotherapy selenium is also been successfully employed in the fight against lymphoedema.*

Everybody, regardless if sick or healthy, should ensure they have a high selenium level, which isn't difficult. A very easy and economic method is buying (unsalted) Brazil nuts. Eating three Brazil nuts a day increased my selenium level to the desired upper limit within just a few weeks.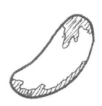

Coconuts or coconut flakes, too, quickly raise selenium levels in the blood. Buying expensive selenium products at the chemist's is therefore unnecessary.

I recommend having selenium levels checked at every blood test as it very much depends on the individual's diet and can thus be easily adjusted. The value should fall within the upper limit of the specified reference range. One also has to bear in mind that a cancer patient needs higher amounts of selenium than a healthy person.

Vitamin D

Vitamin D is not a vitamin in the proper sense of the word but a hormone and is essential for every single body cell. The skin naturally creates vitamin D through ultraviolet sunlight. To date its positive influence has been established for roughly 20 different kinds of tumours. Vitamin D suppresses the tumour's growth, reduces the generation of new vessels to feed the tumour and weakens the signals to trigger growth and metastases formation.

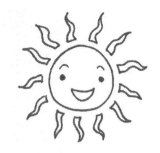

Vitamin D sends increased impulses to the body to prompt the programmed cell death. Quite a number of studies confirm the connection between vitamin D deficiency and several frequent cancer types such as prostate, colon and breast cancer which occur significantly more often where less vitamin D is created in the skin due to low sun exposure. Especially in our latitudes, and particularly during the winter months, people experience a serious lack of vitamin D.

But vitamin D not only aids cancer prevention, it can also keep the degenerated cells in check after the outbreak of the disease. In 2008 scientists in Toronto conducted a study with 512 women who had had breast cancer surgery and whose vitamin D levels had been regularly checked over a ten year period. They found that for women with low vitamin D levels, the likelihood of metastases formation was 94 percent higher than for those with sufficient vitamin D supplies.

Vitamin D levels can be increased by:
- *Sunbathing*: ideally three to four times weekly for about 30 minutes each. Exposing face and hands to the sun is sufficient.
  In the summer I try to enjoy the sun for at least 20 minutes every day, preferably in the morning and without applying sunscreen. This lets me naturally absorb a high amount of vitamin D. Only then do I use a high-quality sun cream whose protection factor corresponds to my skin type.

- *Solarium:* UVB radiation with a wavelength of 280-320 nm.
  Here, too, one has to be careful not to overstrain the skin.
- *Diet:* cod liver oil, salmon, herrings, trout, sardines, tuna and mackerel all contain natural vitamin D, but not enough to satisfy the daily requirement.
- *Dietary supplements:* vitamin D capsules/drops – the recommended dosage differs. In the winter I take one 5000 IU capsule nearly every day. To be on the safe side, the correct dosage should be discussed with a medical professional and regularly checked through blood tests.

Every day for nearly two years I had to take cortisone due to a necrosis as a side effect of my radiotherapy. During that time I tried to maintain my vitamin D level with a vitamin D_3 derivative containing the active ingredient alfacalcidol.

There are various types of vitamin D. Only vitamin D_2 and vitamin D_3, however, are important for the human metabolism. Vitamin D_2 (ergocalciferol) is synthesised from plants and can be ingested by eating plant-based foods. Vitamin D_3 (cholecalciferol), on the other hand, is generated in the skin by the body itself through the sun's UVB radiation. It can also be found in certain animal products and therefore also ingested through one's diet. However, both forms of vitamin D are not effective in the body until they have been converted in the liver and kidney into 1.25-dihydroxyvitamin D, its biologically active form. This activated D hormone, also called calcitriol, achieves the typical effects generally ascribed to vitamin D. But sometimes the conversion of vitamin D into its active form can be interrupted or impeded in the kidney. Here no positive results can be achieved by a diet rich in vitamin D or food supplements like vitamin D capsules. In such cases one can revert to taking so-called active vitamin D metabolites (alfacalcidol), as these bypass the conversion process in the kidney.

Using vitamin D metabolites should be discussed with a physician or, ideally, an endocrinologist and monitored through regular calcium level checks.

While I was on cortisone I took these active vitamin D metabolites because I suspected that my body may not have generated and converted sufficient amounts of vitamin D due to the cortisone. Currently, I have my vitamin D level in the blood measured twice a year and ensure that it is within the upper range.

Vitamin K

One of the long-term side effects of radiotherapy in the head area can also be a radiation necrosis with bone resorption in the sensitive lower jaw bone. During my research I read reports about dissolving, porous (brittle) bones, so I searched for food supplements which can counteract bone resorption. Besides the already mentioned vitamin D and potassium, magnesium and calcium (generally known as beneficial for maintaining healthy bones), vitamin K is another highly important substance.

It exists in various forms of which vitamin K_1 and vitamin K_2 are vital for the human metabolism. Vitamin K_1 originates from plants and is mainly found in green-leafed vegetables, algae and vegetable oils. The most high-yield vitamin K_2 source (MK-7) is natto, a fermented Japanese soya bean product.

Vitamin D_3 and vitamin K_2 work closely together, as vitamin D facilitates increased calcium absorption from food, while vitamin K_2 ensures that calcium is actually stored where it is needed in the body, in the bones and teeth, for instance.

Although vitamin K_2 is partly generated by bacteria in

the human colon, it occurs so rarely in our diet, I decided to take it in its most effective natural form - menaquinone (MK-7).

Because vitamin K_2 can be more easily absorbed through the intestine than vitamin K_1, it is more effective for healthy bones.

Vitamin K_2 (MK-7) in combination with, potassium, magnesium, calcium from our diet and omega-3 oils generates a "power-bone-package".

It has also been established that K_2 possesses anticarcinogenic properties. A study showed the risk of developing cancer decreased the higher the daily vitamin K_2 dosage.

It has also been shown that the risk of prostate carcinomas is enormously reduced the more vitamin K_2 levels increase.

Caution: Vitamin K can weaken the effect of blood-thinning medication.

Secondary plant substances

The umbrella term "secondary plant substances" encompasses a group of chemically very different substances. These are exclusively generated from plants, yet not required by them for energy metabolism or cell structure. The plant mainly utilises them as antibodies against pests and diseases and as growth regulators. Secondary plant substances influence people's food choices through their aroma, taste and colour. They are also said to have various health-promoting benefits.

The secondary plant substances contained in fruit, vegetables, sprouts and seeds play an important part in fighting cancer because they can inhibit the division of cancer cells by obstructing their supply through the blood vessels. In addition they aid the cancer cells' programmed suicide (apoptosis). As such these secondary plant substances, the plant develops for its own protection can also protect humans from diseases.

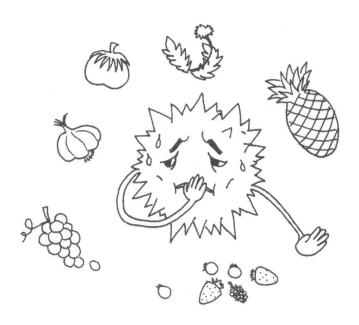

Fig. 18: That's what cancer cells are afraid of – the tumour's growth is inhibited.

Primary plant substances, on the other hand, are those vital to the plant for energy metabolism and cell structure. Our diet usually provides us sufficiently with primary plant substances (proteins, carbohydrates, fats), which also serve to build-up body parts or produce essential energy.

Up-to-date research has discovered more than 10,000 secondary plant substances in edible plants. The most important for the human organism amongst them are:

- *Carotenoids:* the most important in the fight against cancer is beta-carotene. Carotenoids are the natural food colourings in red, yellow and green vegetables.
- *Flavonoids* and *phytoalexins* (polyphenols): nearly all fruit and vegetables contain flavonoids. They are most

widely found in red-coloured plants. Like carotenoid, flavonoids can render free radicals in the body harmless and thus prevent the development of cancer. Phytoalexins are of special importance, particularly the so-called salvestrols, according to Professor Dan Burke. Plants generate phytoalexins for their own protection, against bacteria or fungi, for example. However, if plants are treated with pesticides, they do not develop phytoalexins. For that reason they are primarily found in organic fruit and vegetables and should be eaten in generous quantities.

- *Sulphides:* These lend their taste and smell to onions, garlic, leeks and chives and can also be anticarcinogenic.
- *Glucosinolates:* These stimulate endogenous detoxification and play a substantial part in fighting cancer. They are highly concentrated in all types of cabbage, but also in radishes and cress.

I try to eat health-promoting secondary plant substances on a daily basis. Here I prefer organic fruit and vegetables, ideally locally produced to shorten their transport time and thus harvested when ripe.

Cabbage

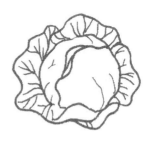

Cabbage is one of the healthiest foodstuffs of all. It is rich in vitamins, minerals, dietary fibres, secondary plant substances and essential oils. All of these endow it with health-promoting and healing properties. Above that, besides calcium, it also contains vitamin C which supports the organism's absorption of calcium.

As cabbage can be eaten, it can be used internally. But it can also be applied externally in the form of a poultice, for example, which can be placed on an area to be treated such as an inflammation.

Because cabbage has detoxifying and anti-inflammatory properties, the American National Cancer Institute (NCI) recommends white cabbage as the leading foodstuff to prevent cancer. Some of its ingredients prohibit the activation of carcinogenic substances.

Other vegetables recommended to prevent cancer include cauliflower, broccoli and Brussels sprouts.

Broccoli

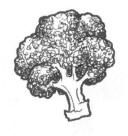

The secondary plant substance sulforaphane, particularly found in broccoli, not only neutralises cancer-causing agents, it apparently also impedes the division of cancer cells. Furthermore it supports the programmed cancer cell death and retards angioneogenesis (the formation of new blood vessels).

Eating broccoli alone does not provide sufficient anticarcinogenic sulforaphane. But it can be supplied by broccoli sprouts which contain 20 to 100 times more glucoraphanin (sulforaphane's precursor). Being aware of the higher concentration of secondary plant substances in broccoli seeds and sprouts, I started growing the seeds and sprouts myself to have the anticarcinogenic substance freshly at my disposal at home. Otherwise one can buy the sprouts in delicatessen shops and sometimes in supermarkets. Some types of sprouts are also available as high dosage tablets or powders.

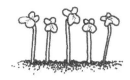

Red berries

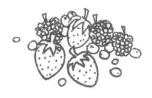

Red berries like raspberries, blueberries and blackberries contain the polyphenol ellagic acid, which severely retards growth factors that create new blood vessels. Thus tumours grow more slowly or stop growing altogether.

I ate tons of fresh raspberries and blueberries especially after my initial diagnosis. They are a delicious addition to muesli in the morning and also a lovely in-between snack. Children love these red berries. My guess is that they may satisfy one of the primal instincts pertaining to a healthy diet.

Scientists at the Hollings Cancer Center at the Medical University of South Carolina verified that ellagic acid impedes the development and spread of cancer far more effectively than most other phenolic acids.

Raspberries, blueberries, strawberries and walnuts contain ellagic acid. As it is highly concentrated in pomegranates, I explored this fruit in more detail.

Pomegranates

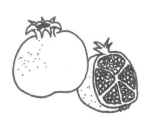

Taking a closer look at the pomegranate one can surmise why Adam let himself be tempted with it by Eve in the Garden of Eden. It is, after all, one of nature's true masterpieces. In its entirety it is far superior to its isolated components, such as ellagic acid, through perfect synergy effects. As such these work in a similar way to antibiotics to fight bacteria, fungi (including Candida) and other parasites and are highly anticarcinogenic.

Similar to red wine, where polyphenols are extracted through fermentation and therefore have a higher concentration than they do in grape juice, pomegranate juice increases the antioxidant and cancer-inhibiting effect through fermentation for the human metabolism. This improves the bioavailability of the pomegranate polyphenols. Bioavailability describes the speed and extent to which a substance is absorbed and its availability where it is needed.

Studies showed the successful use of pomegranates in cancer cells in the breast, pancreas, uterus, prostate, colon, skin, lungs and oesophagus where the tumour's growth was in some cases completely arrested. Research also showed the pomegranate's preventative effect on malign diseases such as prostate and mammary carcinomas.

In addition, pomegranate polyphenols may sensitise tumour cells in preparation for radio- and chemotherapy because they counteract the tumour cells' resistance to their programmed death (apoptosis).

Furthermore, pomegranates contain hormones identical to those in the body and, similar to hormone replacement therapy, can ease menopausal problems.

Its thick skin makes the pomegranate extremely resilient and durable for weeks, even without excessive preservatives. It takes a little practice to quickly and cleanly remove the pips, but the result is well worth it. I often enjoy this wonderful fruit as it is or mixed into a smoothie.

Whenever I don't have the time to freshly prepare it, I use a ready-made, fermented pomegranate concentrate in my muesli or smoothies.

Plant based anticancer agents – salvestrols

As a defence mechanism against pathogens, plants develop special secondary plant substances which can also benefit humans. They are found in the skin of fruit, in the leaves and outer areas of roots and in those parts of the plant which comes into contact with pests such as bacteria, viruses and mould fungi. These defence substances, also called salvestrols, however, only develop in plants which are not treated with chemicals. Plants which have been sprayed don't have to protect themselves by generating salvestrol, and therefore don't produce the healthy secondary plant substance.

Professor Dan Burke and his team at the University of Aberdeen discovered an enzyme called CYP1B1 in tumour cells. Numerous subsequent trials established that this enzyme can act against the tumour cell once it is activated by a "partner". This partner turned out to be salvestrol.

Salvestrols are all those secondary plant substances or antioxidants that can activate the CYP1B1 enzyme, regardless of their chemical composition.

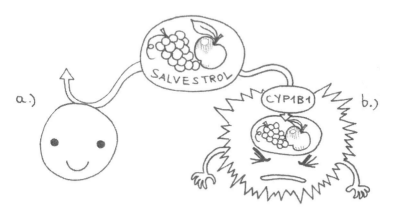

Fig. 19: a.) The salvestrol molecule leaves the benign cell without damaging it.
b.) The salvestrol molecule penetrates the cancer cell and activates the CYP1B1 enzyme.

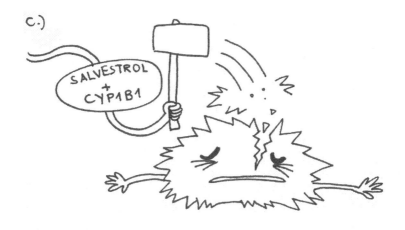

c.)

Fig. 19: c.) For the cancer cell a fatal toxin is going to be created.

A salvestrol molecule enters the cancer cell via the bloodstream. The enzyme CYP1B1 inside the cancer cell combines with the salvestrol molecule and is converted into a deadly toxin.

Organically grown plants such as apples, asparagus, artichokes, olives, pumpkins, redcurrants, strawberries, dandelions and milk thistle contain these salvestrols.

Successful results have been detected in cancer patients suffering from lung, breast, bladder and prostate cancer and melanomas.

To treat cancer, the salvestrol required exceeds at least ten times the amount found in a normal diet. It is therefore advisable to take it as a food supplement. Cancer patients are frequently administered as much as 200 times stronger dosage than the usually daily dose taken in through food.

There are salvestrols in capsule form which are preferable for use in therapeutic treatment.

Salvestrols should not be taken in conjunction with vitamin B17, as the vitamin obstructs their effect.

Personally, I repeatedly take a capsule with a 2000 point content (the unit in which the salvestrol content is measured) separately to other dietary supplements.

White, green and black tea

White, green and black tea all derive from the Camellia sinensis shrub. The biggest difference between the three types is the degree of fermentation.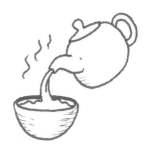

White tea has a minimal degree and is thus the most natural in terms of processing. *Green tea* is largely unfermented because the immediate roasting of the freshly harvested leaves deactivates the enzymes responsible for fermentation within seconds. In the case of *black tea*, however, the leaves are first left to wilt and the enzymes responsible for fermentation (polyphenol oxidase) are released. Subsequently rolling the tea leaves, which breaks open their cells, leads to fermentation. During this course the polyphenols are converted into black pigments. After that the leaves are roasted, thereby ending the fermentation process.

Due to the strong fermentation and the associated low proportion of anticarcinogenic agents, black tea plays no part in cancer treatment.

There are numerous types of green and white teas of varying quality and effect.

Because the area of cultivation, the time of harvesting and processing influences the active ingredients in tea, it makes sense to drink green and white teas from different biological growing areas.

I had known for quite some time that green tea was supposed to possess many healthy ingredients. But I only realised how it exactly affects our health and that it even has anticarcinogenic properties during my stay in Japan.

The Japanese have tea ceremonies which revolve around the preparation of green tea, mainly using the finely ground leaves, known as matcha. I also became enthusiastic about green tea and drank large amounts of all sorts of it, ground or prepared from leaves.

By now some coffee house chains have discovered green tea as well and offer it in addition to their usual product range.

Green tea contains more than 2000 known polyphenols (secondary plant substances) in extremely rich and complex structures. Polyphenols regulate plant growth and repel diseases and parasites. One of the polyphenol subgroups are catechins, also referred to as flavanols. They are considered to be the most important group of health-promoting polyphenols found in tea. Here, in turn, the catechin EGCG (epigallocatechin gallate) constitutes one of the most important ingredients of green tea. About three cups of green tea distribute enough EGCG to the organism for it to block certain cell-receptor signals which would otherwise let cancer cells invade foreign tissue. Furthermore, EGCG can obstruct receptors in the cells that send out the signal for the formation of new blood vessels.

It appears that green tea has a preventative and inhibiting effect on cancer on various levels and supposedly protects the body from lung, stomach, colon and breast cancer and others, as well as counteracting the growth of intestinal tumours, leukaemia, breast, prostate and renal cancer. Because green tea blocks the tumour cells' supply of blood vessels, it seems that it generally prevents the disease from developing.

In order to ensure the catechins' best possible release, the tea should draw for ten minutes and drunk within an hour before the polyphenols evaporate.

Whenever I don't have the time to make green or white tea, I take a capsule of green tea extract.

Dandelion and dandelion root powder

Again I wondered about other (as yet unknown) miracle cures for cancer. Then I asked myself why we always look for the fanciest solutions and believe that rare exotic plants can heal us. Why don't we search for a strong indigenous plant instead? I thought about all the dandelions which proliferate wildly in our garden and would have long gotten out of hand if I wouldn't keep digging it up with its roots. I instantly started researching on the internet and found a number of clinical studies which verified the anticarcinogenic effect of dandelion leaves and dandelion root extract.

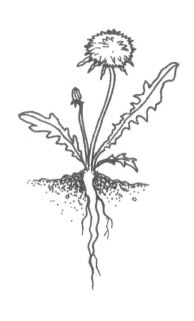

According to one of these studies conducted in 2008, dandelion leaf extracts can inhibit the growth of breast cancer cells. Another study showed that the dandelion root extracts can initiate a "suicide programme" in leukaemia cells which triggers apoptosis, the pre-programmed cell death. In a study published in 2011, dandelion root extracts were even shown to introduce cell death in human melanoma cells (skin cancer cells) without the healthy cells being damaged.

For me dandelion roots are very bitter, but bitter compounds, amongst others, are essential in our diet and nowadays mostly missing from it. Although I didn't regularly take the powder, I am convinced that it may well be worth trying.

I use dandelion leaves in salads, smoothies and my home-made herbal salt.

Because both the leaves and the roots have their effects, it would be advisable to incorporate the whole plant in one's diet. Of course, dandelion root powder, dandelion leaves or dandelion juice are also commercially available and do not necessarily have to be made at home.

Products derived from dandelions can support cancer treatment as non-toxic therapeutic agents and even help in the case of drug-resistant cancer types. Their use should, however, be discussed with the attending physician.

Anticarcinogenic herbs and spices

The flavonoids contained in certain herbs also obstruct the formation of new blood vessels, thus hampering cancer cell proliferation. Anticarcinogenic herbs and spices include rosemary, oregano, basil, mint, thyme, marjoram, parsley, celery, garlic, onions, leeks and chives.

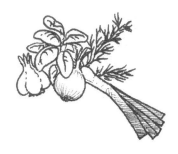

It is easy to incorporate many of them into ones daily diet. I frequently like cooking with garlic and onions, I use basil, parsley and chives on a piece of bread with butter or in salads, and I mix some refreshing mint into my smoothies.

Enzymes

Immediately after my radiotherapy a doctor specialising in complimentary cancer treatments recommended an enzyme mixture. So I investigated the importance of enzymes for the human organism.

Enzymes are vital protein molecules which are basically involved in all metabolic processes. Without enzymes we couldn't live. I would therefore like to explain them in more detail with regard to three main fields of activity they assume in our body: metabolic enzymes, digestive enzymes and food enzymes.

Metabolic enzymes are produced in the cells and are everywhere in the body. They maintain the brain, heart, kidney and lung functions, but are also present in the bones, the blood and the cells themselves.

Digestive enzymes are secreted by the salivary glands, the stomach, the pancreas and the small intestine and help to break down food components.

As such enzymes aid the break-down of the molecular building blocks: carbohydrates into glucose, fats into glycerine and fatty acids, proteins into amino acids.

Food enzymes are found in fresh, raw, uncooked food-stuffs. They fulfil the same function as digestive enzymes, i.e. breaking the food down into its components so it can be absorbed by the bloodstream. When food is heated to roughly more than 45 °C (113 °Fahrenheit) or deep-frozen, its enzyme activities decrease dramatically and no longer assist digestion. To support the body during the digestive process one should therefore include fresh, raw foods rich in enzymes, be it as a side salad, vegetables or fruit, in one's diet. Chewing also helps to "conserve" digestive enzymes. Whenever the body does not receive sufficient amounts of food enzymes, it has to use its energy to generate more digestive enzymes. This energy is then missing elsewhere as in the repair of damaged tissue, for example.

Enzymes themselves don't exhaust themselves during their work, but every protein's lifespan is limited and therefore also that of the enzymes. Once an enzyme becomes too old, it is "split" by a young, healthy enzyme and dissolved.

The new enzyme now takes over its function wherever it is needed and activated by the body. Activating some enzymes requires coenzymes, also called helper molecules. A widely known coenzyme is Q10 (CoQ10) which will be described in more detail later.

However, coenzymes dissipate themselves and need constant renewal. For the body to generate these important helper molecules it needs vitamins (A, B, C, E and K), minerals (magnesium, sodium and potassium) as well as trace elements (copper, manganese, iron, zinc and selenium). The list alone shows how important it is to ensure the body is sufficiently supplied with natural vitamins, minerals and trace elements.

People who eat little raw food can develop an enzyme deficiency and subsequently be more prone to diseases. Enzymes support the body in overcoming pathogens and damaging influences and also help to prevent acute inflammations becoming chronic. In conventional treatment enzyme mixtures are often used alongside the tumour therapy. Most used are proteolytic enzymes which break the protein down into smaller units. Enzyme mixtures applied in cancer treatment improve the blood flow and are thus intended to impede the settlement of cancerous daughter cells and the formation of metastases. Enzymes can also destroy the cancer cells' protective layer, thereby enabling white blood cells to attack the cancer cells. Enzyme preparations should be taken with lots of water on an empty stomach at least half an hour before meals.

If food is eaten too hot, enzyme systems can be destroyed in the stomach lining. One should generally not eat or drink anything too hot as this can cause chronic internal burns, resulting in inflammations. It is therefore hardly surprising that consuming excessively hot food is associated with higher incidences of throat, tongue, oesophagus and stomach cancer. Because by now I understand the connection between disease and chronic inflammation, I follow my grandmother's advice that a drink only has the correct temperature when you can immerse the tip of your finger in it for five seconds without feeling pain.

Following my radiotherapy I took an enzyme mixture (in capsule form) consisting of: papain, bromelain, amylase, lipase, trypsin, α-chymotripsin, L-glutathione, rutin and thymus substance for several months.

Coenzyme Q10

In a simplified way a coenzyme can be described as an enzyme's partner who helps it doing its job. The coenzyme Q10 (CoQ10) is a vital, fat-soluble molecule found in nearly every body cell. It helps the cells to convert nutrition into energy-rich molecules. One could call it the spark that triggers energy production. More than that it is also a strong antioxidant and thus catches free radicals.

CoQ10 mainly exists in two forms: oxidised (ubiquinone), or reduced (ubiquinol).

The overall CoQ10 level in the organism decreases with advanced age and also through severe illnesses, as does the body's ability to convert the CoQ10 (ubiquinone) into ubiquinol, its bioactive antioxidant form.

The intestine absorbs ubiquinol close to ten times more easily than ubiquinone. It is therefore far easier on the system to use the CoQ10's active form ubiquinol. Scientific reports indicate that a massive reduction of the ubiquinol level and increased oxidative stress facilitates many age-related illnesses, but also cardiovascular diseases and cancer.

Amongst other foods, ubiquinol is found in nuts, onions, potatoes, cauliflower, broccoli, eggs and cold-pressed oils.

A CoQ10 deficit can be counteracted by taking ubiquinone or, even better ubiquinol (as drops or tablets).

Bitter substances – the forgotten taste

Bitter substances are chemical compounds with a bitter taste. Plants develop them as defence mechanisms against predators. They are often found in nature, amongst other plants in dandelions, yarrow or common centaury.

Bitter substances stimulate our digestive organs and take effect as soon as they touch the tongue. Their bitter taste stimulates the gall bladder, the stomach, the liver and pancreas, thereby releasing bile, gastric juices and insulin. Sadly the bitter taste has been bred out of many natural foods over the last decades. I only realised how important they are when I studied the dietary habits of the world's oldest people. My research concluded that there are several countries where people increasingly live to an above average age. These included the Hunzukuc people in Pakistan. So I asked myself what contributed to their old age.

For a long time the Hunzukuc were isolated in the not easily accessible Hunzukuc valley and were known to frequently live over a 100, enjoying the best quality of life. Until a road leading into the valley was built, bringing with it the associated lifestyle changes, these people didn't suffer from any kind of cancer. Several doctors who had made the difficult journey into the Hunzukuc valley since the beginning of 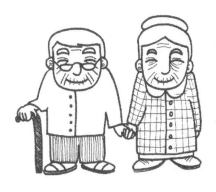 the 20th century reported this fact. They described how the Hunzukuc people's diet consisted mainly of apricots, apricot seeds and apricot oil as well as cereals and fresh vegetables. The Hunzukuc and other cancer-free peoples' longevity and vitality is generally attributed to favourable factors such as plenty of exercise in the fresh air and sun, eating in moderation and a mainly fruit and vegetable diet. These people not only eat natural foods, they also consume the most varied types of fruit including the seeds and pips,  most of which have a high proportion of bitter substances.

These contain cyanide compounds called nitriles. So I informed myself about bitter substances, particularly amygdalin, also referred to as vitamin B17, and made an interesting discovery.

"Vitamin" B17 – amygdalin – laetrile

As per definition vitamin B17, is not a vitamin because it is not essential for the human metabolism. Yet the term is widely used. It's also known as amygdalin and laetrile.

More so than any other biological cancer treatment, vitamin B17 has provoked controversial views and even bitter feuds amongst the experts. Numerous medical professionals around the world (Andreas Puttich, Manuel Navarro, Shigeaki Sakai and many more) reported and still report that a large number of cancer patients have been successfully treated with vitamin B17. Others, however, condemn it as toxic, even deadly.

Caught between the varying views I started searching the net for first-hand patient accounts and was surprised by 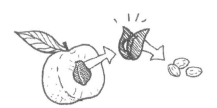 the amount of positive feedback from people who take vitamin B17 in the form of the apricot's bitter, soft inner kernel.

They usually start with one to two kernels a day, but it is frequently increased up to 40 kernels a day over the course of a month. These include cancer patients of my own acquaintance and they are doing well.

The vitamin B17 molecule consists of two sugar molecules (glucose), one cyanide molecule (hydrocyanic acid) and one benzaldehyde molecule (artificial bitter almond oil). According to the B17 proponents, this combination inside its molecule is not toxic for humans although it is composed of cyanide and benzaldehyde, both of them are definitely toxic in isolation. In their opinion the stable B17 molecule can only be "cracked" by the beta-glucosidase enzyme (splitting enzyme).

Beta-glucosidase is abundantly present where cancer cells have formed. Because vitamin B17 also contains two sugar molecules besides cyanide and benzaldehyde, the cancer cell greedily jumps at the sugar and "inadvertently" splits the stable B17 molecule in the process. A fatal indulgence for the cancer cells as they also snack on the toxins.

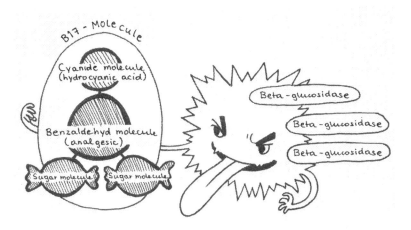

Fig. 20: Cancer cells are greedy and split the B17 molecule with the help of beta-glucosidase.

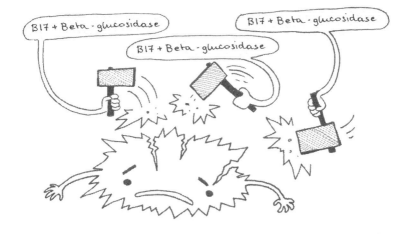

Fig. 21: Vitamin B17 and beta-glucosidase release deadly toxins which destroy the cancer cell.

Healthy cells contain another enzyme called rhodanese which can convert cyanide into thiocyanate. Thiocyanate supposedly has extremely health-promoting properties, though nowadays it is usually not sufficiently supplied in people's diets, which has too little raw food or/and too many processed foods. In healthy cells, toxic benzaldehyde is converted to pain-relieving benzoic acid with the aid of atmospheric oxygen. Cancer cells, on the other hand, which don't feed their metabolism with oxygen but through anaerobic digestion, don't stand a chance against benzaldehyde. A 2014 article published by Frankfurt's Goethe University in collaboration with the University of Göttingen, showed a clear growth-retarding effect of B17 on bladder cancer cells.

The effect of vitamin B17 can apparently be further increased through additionally taking enzyme preparations. In this context the pancreatic enzymes trypsin and α-chymotrypsin are of particular importance in cancer treatment. Enzymes are meant to uncover cancer cells and make them

151

attackable through the body's own immune system.

Although the vitamin B17 opponents agree that cyanide is converted into the relatively non-toxic thiocyanate with the aid of the rhodanese enzyme, they are still of the opinion that a fatal dose of hydrocyanic acid for humans is 0.7 mg per kg of bodyweight. A person weighing 70 kg, for instance, would therefore be killed by 49 mg of cyanide releasing hydrocyanic acid.

Because an apricot kernel contains about 0.9 mg of cyanide, 49 mg of cyanide would correspond to roughly 54 kernels. However, one has to bear in mind that nature can also show fluctuations. But I do want to point out that various authorities warn about the consumption of foodstuffs containing amygdalin. With regard to apricot kernels they recommend a maximum consumption of two per day or none at all.

Bitter apricot kernels also contain B vitamins (B_1 to B_9), C and E vitamins and minerals including potassium, calcium, magnesium and phosphor. Furthermore apricot kernels are rich in amino acids such as arginine, leucine, glycine and proline as well as trace elements like iron, zinc, manganese and copper.

Before my treatment in Japan I received vitamin B17 infusions in Germany without any side effects. Vitamin B17 infusions are still used by many medical and alternative practitioners including practitioners in Germany.

In Austria the use of vitamin B17 for medical purposes is not allowed. Yet bitter apricot kernels are also available here. The Contreras Clinic in Tijuana, Mexico, ensures a strict diet in conjunction with administering vitamin B17 (which is converted into a highly pure solution using ethanol before being infused). The diet applied more or less corresponds to the principle of "back to nature".

As vitamin B17 is found in an extremely high concentration in bitter apricot kernels, I bought a 1 kg bag of the organic variety. I frequently chew some of them to supply myself with sufficient amounts of bitter substances, preferably together with dried or fresh pineapple (contains bromelain) or papayas (contains papain). I make sure to spread this over the course of my day because I don't want to overtax my body's detoxification processes. At times I combine taking bitter apricot kernels with an enzyme mixture of: papain, bromelain, amylase, lipase, trypsin, α-chymotriypsin, L- glutathione, rutin and thymus substance. After my radiotherapy this enzyme combination was recommended to me by a doctor specialising in complementary cancer therapies.

Although one often reads about cancer being cured through vitamin B17 alone, I believe this to be the exception. Overall, however, I suspect that vitamin B17 can play a vital part after conventional treatment.

Be that as it may, anyone interested in taking it should be sufficiently informed and, if necessary, consult a practitioner of natural therapies.

The value of whole grain

While researching healthy nutrition I often read about the importance of wholemeal products. So I took a closer look at the composition of a grain kernel. It mainly consists of four parts:
- Bran (fruit and seed coats)
- Germ
- Endosperm
- Aleurone layer

Bran contains a large part of the grain's minerals and most of its roughage.

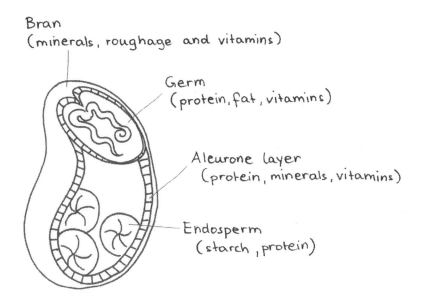

Bran
(minerals, roughage and vitamins)

Germ
(protein, fat, vitamins)

Aleurone layer
(protein, minerals, vitamins)

Endosperm
(starch, protein)

Fig. 22: Composition of a grain kernel.

The *germ* is the "embryo" of the future plant. Its cells are rich in fat, protein and vitamins.

The *endosperm* forms the largest part of the grain kernel. It contains nearly all of its starch, but hardly any minerals or dietary fibres. The protein in the endosperm is called gluten and important for the flour's baking properties. The endosperm is covered by the *aleurone layer* which predominantly contains high-quality protein, vitamins, minerals and dietary fibres.

When corn is ground into flour there are several possibilities. Maximum separation of bran and endosperm results in white flour with lots of starch and gluten quality suitable for baking bread rolls, for instance. If the separation is not quite as strict, we get darker types of flour with a higher proportion of minerals and roughage. The whole grain is used for wholemeal flour, therefore the most valuable of flour types. When producing white flour the discarded bran and germ yield a by-product collectively called bran. As can be seen in Figure 22 depicting the composition of grain, they are particularly rich in minerals, protein, fat and dietary fibres. For that reason bran has always been used as a species-appropriate, high quality animal feed. Would we give them the endosperm instead, they would not survive for very long.

Eating products made from white flour means we only ingest the grain's inferior part.

Freshly ground wholemeal flour cannot be stored for a long time. The also ground germ is high in fats and quickly turns rancid. One should only buy organically grown whole grains and freshly ground them into flour in one's own flour mill shortly before use.

Omega-3 and omega-6-fatty acids – the secret lies in the proportion

Modifications in foods such as milk, eggs and meat came about through a change in livestock farming and require us to rethink our dietary habits.

It is no secret that the fruit and vegetables we eat no longer yield the same vitamin contents they used to, partly due to mass production, premature harvesting, fertilisers, preservation and cultivation. What is, however, relatively unknown is the fact that milk and meat products from intensive livestock farming have greatly changed in their composition. This particularly applies to the fatty acid content of substances such as omega-3 and omega-6.

According to estimates the ratio of omega-3 to omega-6 fatty acids in the diet of prehistoric people was approx. 1:2. Today the proportion shows an imbalance of up to 1:20 in favour of omega-6 fatty acid.

Our health largely depends on the balance between omega-3 and omega-6, and therefore it is important to ensure that the balance between the two fatty acids is not too big. A proportion of no more than 1:5 is considered advisable.

Milk products from cattle exclusively fed with green fodder show a balanced omega-3 to omega-6 ratio. Once part of this is replaced with grain or soya the omega-3 proportion is drastically reduced as both soya and grains contain a high amount of omega-6. The same applies to the eggs produced by hens without proper animal welfare.

But there's another reason one should use milk and milk products with caution. According to a study conducted by Harvard University, industrially produced dairy products are potential carcinogens in view of their hormone content. This is related to the fact that cows are milked up to 300 days of the year to fully exploit their "milk yield", even when they are in calf. But the more the cow's pregnancy advances, the higher the hormone levels in its milk. The subsequent high levels of the oestrogen compound estrone sulphate is suspected of promoting hormone-induced cancers such as testicular, prostate and breast cancer. For this reason dairy products should be consumed in moderation and only from non-pregnant, pasture-grazing cows. I wish the dairy industry would react appropriately and introduce specific markings to indicate this.

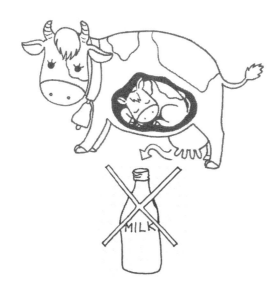

An imbalance between omega-3 and omega-6 fatty acids is proinflammatory as a surplus of omega-6 fatty acids is first converted into arachidonic acid and then into prostaglandins (tissue hormones) with a proinflammatory effect through metabolic processes in the organism. This increases the risk of heart and vascular disease as well as all inflammatory diseases and cancer.

Compensating for an omega-3 fatty acid deficiency is therefore paramount.

Amongst other things this can be achieved by exclusively consuming meat and dairy products from pasture-raised animals. The label that products derive from organic farms is not enough.

A highly effective way of adjusting the imbalance between omega-6 and omega-3 fatty acids is taking oils whose proportion of omega-3 fatty acids exceeds that of omega-6 fatty acids. Oils from plant sources with a particularly high proportion of essential alpha-linolenic acids include the indigenous linseed oil as well as the two exotic chia and perilla oils. The most important of the oils from animal sources to compensate for a deficit of omega-3 fatty acids is krill oil.

Linseed oil

Linseed oil is obtained from the flax plant. Basically one should only consume its organic, cold-pressed variety.

Its anti-inflammatory properties also impede the development of certain cancers.

I have made a habit of having muesli with freshly ground linseed, curd, linseed oil and fresh fruit for breakfast. A variation of this basic combination is the addition of browntop millet, oat flakes, nuts, ground tigernuts, spelt bran, coconut flakes, psyllium husks, even preserved elderberries, chia seeds, broccoli sprouts and so on. Especially at the start of adjusting to a brand-new diet, all this can amazingly influence one's digestion. I also noticed a dramatic improvement in my eyesight. My hairdresser actually commented on the improved quality of my hair. I partially attribute this to taking linseed oil. It is also one of the fatty acids with an especially high level of unsaturated fats; it regulates the acid-alkaline balance and is of particular importance for the human brain function.

But be careful: Linseed oil is an extremely vulnerable unsaturated oil and quickly oxidises when being exposed to atmospheric oxygen. It should always be stored in a cool place, but can also be kept in the freezer for several weeks without solidifying and losing its taste due to its low melting point of approx. -18 °C.

Because of its light sensitivity, I always store linseed oil in a dark bottle and use it up within a maximum of two months to preserve its quality and taste.

Krill oil can be substituted for the already mentioned plant oils. It is derived from crustaceans and is also an excellent source of omega-3.

Krill oil

Krill are small crabs at the very bottom of the food-chain. The name krill derives from the Norwegian and loosely translated means whale food. These small crustaceans feed on phytoplankton and are therefore largely free from heavy metals and pesticides.

Krill oil contains the two essential fatty acids EPA (eicosapentaenoic acid) and DHA (docosahexaenoic acid). Linseed, on the other hand contains both of these fatty acids' precursor, alpha-linolic acid (ALA), which the body still has to convert to EPA and DHA through enzyme action. Krill oil is therefore easier on the body because it already contains the essential fatty acids EPA and DHA.

Taking krill oil protects the cell membranes particularly well from cancer, degeneration and ageing.

Like linseed oil, krill oil is also an anti-inflammatory adversary of our diet which usually contains a surplus of omega-6 fatty acids. People with a high proportion of omega-3 fatty acids in their diet, suffer far more rarely from cancer types like prostate, breast, colon, skin and pancreatic cancer.

Small fish, big fish

For a long time I believed that fish, no matter how large or small, is good for us and supplies valuable omega-3.

On the supermarket shelves smoked salmon is frequently advertised as having a high proportion of omega-3, which it does. What is largely unknown, though, is that salmon all over the world is highly polluted with heavy metals. Other types of fish also contain large amounts of environmental toxins. The reason why is simple and sad, we humans increasingly pollute our oceans. The bigger the fish (i.e. closer to the top of the food chain), the more "contaminated" they are. Large animals like polar bears, for instance, which predominantly feed on big fish and seals, are still extremely contaminated despite their otherwise clean environment. The toxin concentration is even higher in fish with a large fat content because fat stores poisons particularly well. Those who value their health should therefore choose small fish which are low in fat and less polluted.

Many carcinogenic toxins also accumulate in human body fat. This leads to an increase in cancer types which present in the adipose tissue or in organs surrounded by it. The most prominent of these are prostate carcinomas and breast cancer. To prevent cancer it is therefore advisable to ensure a low body fat percentage.

Human beings, who are also at the top of the food chain, should eat food which is as low in harmful substances as possible and regularly detoxify if they want to live a healthy, long life.

For a long time I didn't realise that we are exposed to a huge amount of poisons every day. Some of these are less dangerous because our body can cope with them. Others, however, can cause serious illnesses.

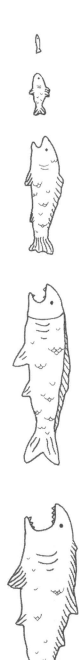

How to remove toxins from the body

Toxins can occur in our food (i.e. heavy metals in fish, antibiotics in meat, pesticides in fruit and vegetables), but also in drinks (i.e. acetaldehyde in plastic bottles) or in the air (i.e. fine dust particles). Curious to find out how the human organism deals with being constantly confronted with these poisons, I examined the body's main detoxifying options more closely.

The liver

The liver provides the most important metabolic functions and is one of the body's most vital detoxification organs. Besides numerous other crucial tasks, for example filtering harmful substances from the blood in the gastrointestinal tract, the liver also filters out old or damaged cells. Unwanted and damaging substances are rendered harmless and excreted through the faeces or the urine. After radiotherapy my liver had to perform an extremely large amount of detoxification. To help it along I took milk thistle capsules. Milk thistle is considered to be the most gentle medicine for the liver. It supports its regeneration process, especially in the case of damages caused by medication.

The liver function can be aided by applying a warm, damp compress. Wrap a hot water bottle in a damp linen cloth and place it on your stomach below the right rib cage. Covered with a dry towel and a cosy blanket, you should now let the compress work for about an hour.

The kidneys

Draining toxins through the kidneys requires a sufficient fluid supply as they also filter the blood and relieve us of harmful substances, which can be excreted through the urine. During radiotherapy, I therefore, meticulously made sure to drink at least three litres of water or unsweetened herbal tea a day. I found a tea blend of wild mallow leaves, nettles and bay leaves particularly beneficial. The complete lack of nausea during my radiotherapy I ascribe to the nettles' detoxifying effect. Drinking large amounts of green tea (an antioxidant as well) I believe also contributed towards my wellbeing during the treatment.

The skin

The skin is an incredibly versatile organ and can secrete certain substances through its sweat glands although to a significantly lower extent than the liver or the kidneys. It is important not to clog its main pores with creams. Regularly brushing the skin with a dry, soft brush and occasional visits to the sauna with moderate but not too hot temperatures (think of your kidneys and make sure you drink enough!) will support its functions.

The gut

The gut absorbs all essential nutrients and excretes "waste". A diet rich in fibres supports the guts function and reduces the risk of food being kept for too long in the intestines.

People who react to gluten-rich foods with constipation or diarrhoea should switch to gluten-free grain varieties such as maize, millet, rice, quinoa, buckwheat or amaranth.

The oral mucosa
(mucous membrane of the mouth)

Daily detoxing via the oral mucosa through oil pulling is simple. Best suited are high-grade organic oils like coconut, linseed or black cumin seed oil. Take a tablespoon of oil, preferably in the morning on an empty stomach, and swirl it around in the mouth for about 10 to 15 minutes. Make sure to spit out all of the whitish mixture of oil, saliva, toxins and bacteria afterwards.

Water is not only the elixir of life, it is also essential for the detoxification process. I therefore start the day with a glass of warm water. 1.5 to 2 litres of it a day help the body to release accumulated toxins.

In addition, eating certain foods (dandelions, artichokes, garlic or parsley for example) and taking specific food supplements (for instance milk thistle) can aid detoxification.

When consciously detoxifying the body, it is particularly important that the toxins are quickly purged from the system. Chlorella algae can bind pollutants and toxins and is then excreted with the faeces or the urine. Over a period of several months I took circa four chlorella capsules a day. The first few days I felt a burning sensation when passing urine which I took to be an obvious reaction to the powerful detoxification. Furthermore I support my body for years now by curcumin and medicinal mushrooms. (See "Medicinal mushrooms", p. 165.)

> **Warning:** *People with dental amalgams who do not suffer from acute cancer should have the amalgam removed before detoxing and then have the body professionally purged from toxins, with chlorella algae, for example. In the case of acute cancer, I recommend preliminarily leaving the amalgam in the teeth so as not to additionally stress the body through the removal.*

Regularly detoxing is important, but it is just as important for the body to reduce its toxin intake:

- As far as possible, I buy organic food, preferably locally farmed. It is still essential to thoroughly wash the produce before consumption. One can generally assume that thick-skinned fruit (such as pomegranates or bananas) is naturally better protected against parasites and should therefore be less polluted with pesticides (Can pesticides be avoided by eating organic products?", 64).

- I try to be careful when it comes to what my body touches and ensure that my soaps, detergents, cleaning agents, deodorants and clothes are as skin-friendly as possible. Health-damaging products and ingredients such as fabric softeners, dyes and aluminium I largely avoid.

- I try to stay in an unpolluted environment and to exercise in fresh air. Since my cancer diagnosis I don't frequent smoky bars. Interestingly enough, I don't just find the smoke unpleasant, it also doesn't agree with me anymore and instantly makes me cough. My reactions are similar in busy streets with high exhaust pollution levels.

Can pesticides be avoided by eating organic products?

In 2002 the scientist Cynthia Curl conducted a study with 39 children aged between two and five to establish if different diets impact on children's pesticide exposure. The children were divided into two groups. The participants of one group consumed predominantly organically produced food while those of the second ate mainly conventionally produced food. Three days later the children's urine was tested for traces of the most common organophosphate pesticides.

The results were conclusive: the pesticide exposure of the children who had eaten organic food was far lower than the statutory limits determined by the US Environmental Protection Agency (EPA) and the pesticide exposure of the children who had largely consumed conventional food was six times higher than the statutory limit.

A study conducted with 13 adults, eleven years later produced a similar result. Here the adults ate primarily organic products for a week, followed by conventional food. The findings confirmed those of Cynthia Curl, an organic diet significantly reduces the body's pesticide exposure.

Thus the answer to the question posed above is a definite "yes". Careful food selection can reduce the pesticide concentration in the system.

Medicinal mushrooms

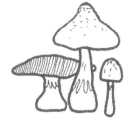

In Japan I noticed a huge variety of mushrooms on the supermarket shelves and observed they are used in numerous dishes. The variety far exceeded that on offer in Austria and aroused my curiosity. When reading up about them, I discovered the effect of medicinal mushrooms.

Many still remember the accident at the Chernobyl nuclear reactor in 1986. People, including my own country's population, were advised not to eat wild mushrooms as they had been radioactively contaminated. Air- and cloud-born, the radioactivity had reached Austria where the rain deposited it on the soil and flora. Fungi absorbed high concentrations of radioactivity when fulfilling their function of detoxifying the environment. Medicinal mushrooms also do this in the human body; hence they are said to possess antibacterial, antiviral, anti-inflammatory and antitumoural properties.

Just like a sponge, medicinal mushrooms can absorb large amounts of toxins and purge them from the body.

Medicinal mushrooms can also help in cases of acute and chronic hyperacidity. The medicinal mushroom, Auricularia, has a de-acidifying effect and quickly eases muscle pain. The Cordyceps mushroom stimulates renal function and increases the basal metabolic rate.

In America and Asia some substances extracted from medicinal mushrooms are officially employed in standard cancer treatments. Medicinal mushrooms have also proven themselves as an addition to chemo- and radiotherapy and can positively influence resilience and overall health. At this stage ten very well researched medicinal mushrooms include: the Coriolus, Hericium, Reishi, Maitake and Shiitake.

The cause for many cancer types has still not been explored, but scientists suspect that the Candida albicans fungus may play a part in it. Amongst other options, it can also be successfully combated with medicinal mushrooms.

Occasionally fungal infections are present after taking antibiotics. I once read that these are more easily healed with the medicinal Coriolus mushroom (within two to three days) than with various ointments or rinses.

Now that I have became even more interested in the subject, researched it in more depth and, fascinated by medicinal mushrooms' many varied uses; I decided to train as a mycotherapist. Some of the mushrooms' areas of application include: high blood pressure, diabetes, allergies, respiratory diseases, bladder infections, hyperacidity, bowel and stomach problems, muscle regeneration, skin diseases and as an addition to cancer therapy. They create an alkaline environment and, most importantly, support the immune system and maintain the white blood cell count. Medicinal mushrooms can, if necessary, be taken right through one's life. They have a homeostatic effect on the body, i.e. they harmonise the metabolism, keep it balanced and set to work wherever the problem is located. I take them in tablet or capsule form and make sure to buy them from verified, reputable suppliers.

What else makes me feel good

Over the following pages I would like to introduce other substances and remedies beneficial to my health, which I take whenever necessary.

Grapefruit seed extract – the plant-based antibiotic

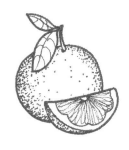

In my eyes, grapefruit seed extract is a wonderful, nearly forgotten, old remedy that belongs in everyone's medicine cupboard. It is obtained from the grapefruit's seeds and juiceless pulp. The desired constituents are extracted with the aid of glycerine.

Grapefruit seed extract has numerous applications because it can fight fungi, viruses and bacteria. Three times 15 drops diluted in water taken daily quickly alleviates the symptoms of colds, coughs, influenza and abdominal influenza. As a natural antibiotic it helps with all infections and inflammations. But, combined with geranium oil, it can also be applied with promising results in the treatment of antibiotic-resistant germs such as MRSA (Methicillin-resistant Staphylococcus aureus) spread in hospitals, which can be particularly fatal to people with a weakened immune system, according to a 2004 study by Manchester Metropolitan University.

Grapefruit seed extract has a fungicidal effect on more than 100 different types of fungi. According to a Polish study, it even has an effect on Candida albicans, which already mentioned, is suspected of being a contributory cancer cause. Grapefruit seed extract may possibly also counteract the intestinal bacterium Helicobacter pylori, which can induce complaints ranging from inflammation of the stomach lining up to stomach cancer.

In my opinion, grapefruit seed extract could possibly also contribute towards cancer prevention.

The body generally easily tolerates grapefruit seed extract and doesn't develop a resistance against it. But in case of a possible, unknown citrus fruit allergy the dose should be carefully administered, starting with one to three drops diluted in water a day and increased to 15 drops three times daily, if it agrees with the body.

To aid the purging of dead bacteria or fungi and their toxins as a result of taking grapefruit seed extract, it is important to drink a lot of fluids, preferably still water.

I also ensure to only buy high-quality, organic grapefruit seed extract.

Warning: Grapefruit products can obstruct a liver enzyme which aids the breakdown of medication. Thus the concentration of pharmaceuticals in the blood can increase many times over and possibly lead to dangerous side effects. This also applies to drugs used during the course of chemotherapy. In this case the body would be inundated with cytotoxins.

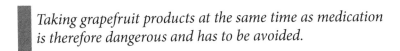

Taking grapefruit products at the same time as medication is therefore dangerous and has to be avoided.

Silicon

Although it is not a "typical anti-cancer drug", I still find it extremely important to ensure a sufficient intake of silicon. It activates cell metabolism and cell structure, improves cell respiration and thus keeps body cells young for a long time.

Above all we need silicon for our skin, nails, hair, bones, joints and elastic connective tissue. Silicon promotes the absorption of calcium and thereby aids bone formation. Moreover, it is even suspected that it binds the calcium in the bones. Millet, oats and barley are excellent sources of silicon. As the long-term side effects of radiotherapy can also be accompanied by local bone resorption in the irradiated area, particularly threatened in this case was the lower jaw bone, it is important to counteract this through sufficient silicon intake.

I sprinkle a tablespoon of oats onto my muesli or mix it into my smoothie every day (100 g of oats contain approx. 425 mg of silicon). This adequately provides me with the valuable trace element.

L-lysine

An acquaintance of mine fought a continuous battle against cold sores. On a pharmacist's recommendation he took six times 500 mg of L-lysine daily for six days to combat the herpes infection when it appeared again, followed by three times 500 mg L-lysine daily as a preventative. His cold sores disappeared after a couple of days and not only that: his nasal mucous membranes, which had tended to bleed very easily for twenty years, regenerated themselves within a few weeks and his chronic sinusitis vanished as well. Impressed by his positive experience, I started to research L-lysine, hoping that it may possibly also be effective in combating cancer, and did actually find reports that L-lysine, in combination with L-proline, green tea and vitamin C, could arrest cancer growth.

L-lysine is an essential amino acid which has to be taken with meals (circa 0.7 to 4 grammes a day, depending on body weight). An insufficient intake of L-lysine can impair immune functions. Amongst other symptoms, tiredness, lack of concentration or dizziness can also indicate an L-lysine deficiency.

Moreover, L-lysine supports intestinal calcium absorption, promotes calcium storage in the bones and can therefore counteract osteoporosis. It is also an essential component of collagen which is found in teeth, bones, tendons, cartilages, ligaments and the skin.

Chicken, beef, Parmesan, milk and eggs are all good sources of L-lysine.

Personally, I repeatedly take L-lysine in capsule form (500 mg/day) over the course of a few weeks and feel the positive effect on my mucous membranes (nose, mouth and throat). I also believe that, amongst other things, it helped to regenerate my cortisone damaged stomach lining.

L-lysine is best taken on an empty stomach early in the morning or late in the afternoon, as *L-arginine* (L-lysine's adversary during protein metabolism) has not yet been absorbed through food intake and L-lysine is thus most effective. Basically the aim is to balance L-lysine and L-arginine, since both are protein building blocks, which are essential for cell structure. In the case of an acute herpes infection or shingles, however, food rich in arginine, such as nuts or wholemeal products, should not be eaten as herpes viruses can only build a protective protein layer through sufficient arginine supply. Some herpes viruses like the Epstein-Barr virus or the human herpesvirus type 8 are directly linked to the development of cancer.

Besides L-lysine, *L-proline* is also significantly involved in the formation of collagen. Collagen, as already mentioned, is an important component of teeth, bones, tendons, cartilages, ligaments and the skin. *L-proline* is a non-essential amino acid which the body can usually produce itself. With prolonged illnesses, however, L-proline's production capacity is frequently depleted and thus insufficient. In these cases additional L-proline should be taken.

Black cumin seed oil

The native Egyptian black cumin plant contains healing substances in poppy seed-like capsules which help to stabilise or build up the immune system. Black cumin seeds were used as far back as ancient Egypt as a cure for colds, toothaches, headaches and inflammations.

The seeds can be eaten or pressed into oil. For therapeutic purposes it is important to use cold-pressed black cumin oil, as the valuable unsaturated fatty acids are destroyed at higher temperatures.

The active agents in black cumin oil can help to combat cancer in several ways by:

- increasing immune cell production,
- protecting the body cells against free radical attacks,
- having an anti-inflammatory effect,
- stimulating the formation of bone marrow cells,
- increasing the number of antibody-producing B cells and
- increasing the production of interferon – a protein which prevents the spread of harmful micro-organisms.

Egyptian black cumin, which grows under optimum climatic conditions, is currently considered to have the highest therapeutic effect.

The power of combination

Foodstuffs or dietary supplements are often more effective when taken in combination than they are on their own.

Combining several "anti-cancer agents" can simultaneously influence a number of mechanisms which play a part in the disease.

Some synergy effects have already been researched, including:

- curcumin, pepper and omega-3 fatty acids
- tomatoes and broccoli
- bitter apricot kernels, pineapple and papaya
- apricot kernel oil and garlic
- linseed oil and curd
- vitamin D, curcumin, pepper and omega-3 fatty acids
- vitamin K_2, vitamin D, omega-3 fatty acids and calcium contained in food
- L-lysine, proline, green tea and vitamin C
- selenium, magnesium, vitamin C and vitamin A

I consciously try to take some of these combinations every day to increase their powerful individual effect even further.

The environment and the immune system

According to a recently published study by the Stanford University School of Medicine, the environment has a much greater impact on our immune system than genetic predisposition (it is estimated that only five to ten percent of all cancers can be ascribed to hereditary factors).

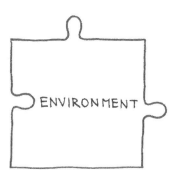

For this reason I try to actively reduce negative external influences on my body:

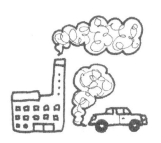

1. As far as possible, I spend my time in an unpolluted environment and try to get plenty of fresh air. Since my diagnosis I avoid smoky bars. It's interesting that I not only find the smoke unpleasant, it also instantly irritates my throat. The same applies to streets where there are excessive exhaust fumes.

2. I pay attention about everything that touches my body and therefore ensure that

the soaps, detergents cleaning agents and deodorants I use and the clothes I wear are as skin-friendly as can be. Additionally I try to avoid fabric softeners, toxic dyes and aluminium.

3. When I need a filling, I ask the dentist to only use plastic or porcelain but never an amalgam.

4. Cooking utensils, fabric dyes or electrosmog can also be harmful. I therefore replace frying pans that have scratched Teflon coating and thoroughly wash new clothes until they no longer, or at least hardly, release any dye. Moreover, I don't keep any electronic appliances close to my sleeping area, I had it checked by a radiesthesia specialist and have subsequently repositioned my bed.

5. Since toxins in the home can be harmful as well, it is advisable to carefully examine all materials used, and, if necessary, replace them with environmentally friendly and compatible products. These include interior wall paints, lacquer on doors, windows and parquet floors as well as chemicals in bed and sofa covers.

Each targeted cancer treatment should be aimed at reducing the absorption of environmental pollutants as far as possible.

The mind influences our immune system

Through personal experience as well as various studies I am aware that the mind can hugely influence cancer. While my tumour had apparently grown extremely slowly for years, which is quite understandable in retrospect considering the gradually emerging symptoms, it started to grow rapidly straight after it's diagnosis.

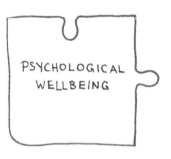

PSYCHOLOGICAL WELLBEING

According to research, isolation, but also fear and permanent stress accompanied by feelings of helplessness, promote cancer development and growth.

A lab experiment with rats conducted by the University of Pennsylvania illustrated how feelings of impotence can massively effect the progression of a disease. Cancer cells with a 50 percent probability of causing a fatal tumour were transplanted into the rats. Then the animals were divided into three groups: the rats in the first group were left to their own devices and, as expected about half of them (54 percent) died within three months. The rats in the second group were helplessly exposed to mild electric shocks. The third group, however, received electric shocks which they could avoid by learning how to press a button.

The results were impressive. Just one month after the start of the experiment 63 percent of the rats who had learned how to avoid the electric shocks were tumour-free, while only 27 percent of those who were helplessly exposed to them had overcome the disease. These findings show that not only stress, per se favours cancer, but the feeling of impotence in situations where we feel helpless.

Negative stressful events provoke inflammatory responses in the body which, in turn, favour cancer. In contrast, positive experiences and feelings of happiness contribute towards a reduction of inflammations in the organism. Particularly interesting is that even pretending to feel emotions like joy and sadness influences the activity of defence cells in the immune system. This was established in a study involving actors. Their defence cells were more active when they acted out cheerful scenes and less active when they acted out negative moods, thus weakening the immune system.

This makes it clear how important it is to train one's mind to be positive, particularly in the case of severe diseases such as cancer.

It frequently takes 10 to 20 years until cancer becomes noticeable and therefore can be detected.

Possible, partly responsible psychological causes can therefore date back a long time.

Essentially cancer seems to me like a distinct lesson on the way back to the self – and beside all the other helpful therapies, probably the most helpful when it comes to unconditionally changing one's life in a way one really wants to live it. Radically and from one day to the next, if needs be.

It is imperative to influence one's health with positive thoughts.

After having been diagnosed with cancer I experienced an all-time low in my psychological wellbeing. I was scared of the unknown, possibly uncontrollable situation I may have had to face.

Today I'm no more and no less afraid of the future than other people. I'm grateful for every day I'm alive and do everything in my power to prevent the disease from recurring. Follow-up examinations mean clarity to me and I'm not worried about them. Occasionally I'm asked what cancer patients most wish for from their relatives. The only answer, in my view is: "adjustable", loving support. At the start it is important to grieve together. Thus the patient feels that they are important to those next to them and would leave a gap if they were no longer there. However, depending on the situation, adjusted support also entails sharing fun and joy besides seriousness. There comes a time when the patient needs diversion and a change of subject. As those around them find it frequently hard to guess what the patient needs at any particular time, especially at the beginning, I recommend to simply ask.

The following ten points illustrate what personally helped me to overcome the psychological low caused by my diagnosis:

- *Letting go*: accepting the "worst case scenario" to combat the fear of possible death. Many years ago I observed a swimming instructor teaching small children. He started by having the children practise immersing their heads in the water. Once they were no longer afraid of this, he showed them swimming movements. When he told them to practise these under or above the water, the children lost their fear of drowning. They now confidently floated on the water and learned how to swim in no time. So whoever loses the fear of drowning can swim. And whoever loses the fear of dying, lays a significant foundation for his life!

- *Informing myself* about my cancer and its possible treatments, as well as, educating myself about anti-carcinogenic diets and dietary supplements, made me feel no longer helpless. Subsequently my feelings of impotence vanished, which positively influenced the healing process.

- Creating a *supportive social environment*. Patients who join appropriate groups have a significantly higher chance of survival.

I therefore started looking for a group of similarly afflicted people. Because my type of cancer (ACC) is relatively rare it was initially difficult to locate such a group for a mutual exchange. Thanks to the internet, however, I eventually found a group in Europe which meets once a year. The closer it came to the date of my first meeting, the more insecure I felt: would this turn out to be a morbid gathering of physically impaired and unhappy people? Would I even be able to cope emotionally? Would it perhaps be better to stay at home after all? But my mother insisted that she'd attend the meeting no matter what and that I could make up my mind to accompany her up to the last minute. I decided to go with her!

Meeting the group

The first meeting took place in the home of a fellow sufferer in a private, cosy atmosphere. The costs involved were also not excessive, which is quite important seeing that most of the participants have travel and accommodation expenses. 15 participants had announced they'd be there, roughly half of them were afflicted and the rest were relatives. As soon as I stepped into the room I was greeted by an unbelievably positive mood. Everyone was in good form and cheerful and we were made feel extremely welcome.

Very soon there was an incredible feeling of closeness among the members of the group, something I had never experienced before with complete strangers in such a short space of time.

It was particularly special for my mother to witness how these cancer patients could be so cheerful, despite such a life changing experience. Up to this point, since I'd been diagnosed, she hadn't really allowed herself to be joyful. As such this meeting was also a significant experience which made her instantly feel better.

The strength and positive, near heroic attitude with which people affected with the disease shape and master their lives is phenomenal. Their heightened awareness of life's finite nature is for some of them, even a downright life-enhancing experience from which their loved ones also profit.

Suddenly I felt no longer isolated with my disease. Instead, I felt we were all in the same boat and thus some very deep emotional friendships developed that I never want to lose.

My only wish to discuss anticarcinogenic diets and dietary supplements with the other members was disappointing. The entire group was of the opinion that our type of cancer (ACC) could not be influenced through diet and/or supplements.

But four years later we were in for a big surprise. By now the group had grown to 35 people. As I still felt as well as I did before and whilst some others unfortunately didn't, interest in me abruptly increased. I was deeply distressed to find that some members were considered to be no longer treatable only a few years after their diagnosis, due to incorrect primary treatment, even though they had been diagnosed after me. In these cases, according to current knowledge, it is hardly ever possible to bring about a positive change. This is one of the main reasons that motivated me to write this book. I want to contribute towards making it easier for sufferers to find the most suitable initial therapy for them, and then to counteract a recurrence of the cancer through an appropriate lifestyle.

Many of the group members now asked what I do to stay healthy.

A further cancer sufferer had joined the group in the meantime. Although she had been diagnosed quite some time ago, the disease hadn't recurred and she was metastasis-free. We therefore discussed our respective "life programmes". They largely corresponded, yet again confirming the benefits of my approach.

I therefore encouraged the group to actively support the immune system. Preferably through a healthy diet and appropriate food supplements, moderate exercise, sufficient sleep and an autonomous, stress-free lifestyle without constantly living in fear if the chosen treatment will work or is working.

Personally I have regular follow-up checks. I'm not scared of them. They will either confirm that I'm healthy or that I can react in time in an emergency!

Since I was diagnosed with cancer I guard my physical strength more sensibly, I don't try to stay awake when I'm tired and more frequently say "no" when I don't like something or if it would be too strenuous for me. I permit myself to be weak every now and then.

Even when successfully treated, cancer has a major impact on people's lives and we should acknowledge and accept its far-reaching effects. At times it also requires changing one's life.

180

- *Having some fun*: As serious as my illness was, I didn't let it dominate my life. I surround myself with people who make me laugh, watch funny movies and visit events that make me feel positive.
- Finding one's *personal key* to combat sadness and tears. My personal key was a fortune teller's absolute conviction a long time ago that I would have children. In the beginning I remembered and clung to this positive thought because children were only an option for me, if I recovered and would see them grow up. My mother was able to stop crying when she read a comment by a cancer sufferer on the internet, which described the impact that he had felt when he had distanced himself from people who wallowed in self-pity, as their attitude didn't promote his wellbeing. Reading this my mother realised that she was crying out of self-pity and had to stop her tears for my sake. From that moment on she felt renewed strength to research my possible treatment options.

  Another cancer patient I had heard of, had found her key when her brother advised her to lock her fears up in a closet and leave them there.

  Everybody has to die. Cancer simply underlines our mortality – let's use this gift of conscious finiteness to live the rest of our lives more purposefully.
- *Shamans and healers* provide optimism and the courage to face life. After my medical diagnosis, doctors mostly looked at me compassionately and made discouraging remarks, which was not really constructive. The first strange people to give me hope were healers and shamans who told me about their own successful fight against cancer. The optimism they instil should not make one reckless, but rather provide the inspiration to be invigorated and optimistic to search for the right conventional medical treatment.
- *Thinking positively*: Actors who acted out happy scenes

consequently had more active defence cells than they had after acting out sad scenes. So we can actually positively influence our mind and therefore our immune system through pretend joy.

- *Looking for closure*: When I decided to investigate the reason for my slight facial nerve paralysis, I consulted a specialist. After visiting this man based on his particular qualifications, following a non-target oriented examination, he fobbed me off with the words: "Let me give you some advice, forget about the whole thing!"
A year and a half after my radiotherapy, I consulted him again because I simply couldn't forget how he had dismissed me before. Had I listened to him or had my mother convinced me to heed his advice, the tumour would have continued to grow and would have cost me my life.

I needed to confront him with his past misdiagnosis. On entering his surgery I asked him if he remembered me. He replied: "Of course, I do." I then probed further to see if he recalled what he had advised me to do. He also answered this in the affirmative. So I told him: "Had I listened to you, I would most probably not be standing here today. You made a fundamental mistake. I did have a malignant tumour."

An awkward silence on the doctor's part.

I elaborated: "Pressure pain and facial paralysis are symptoms of a malignant tumour. This information can be quite easily found on the internet. Why didn't you even consider that possibility? You didn't take me seriously and that very nearly cost me my life! Not everyone looking for advice stays true to his gut feeling when a trained doctor tells him the opposite."

Now the eminent authority sitting in front of me pointed to a substantial volume and elucidated very slowly: "This textbook states that 99 percent of facial paralysis cases are not due to a malignant tumour –

besides you're far too young. "He then asked me what I wanted from him. My reply: "I'm begging you here and now to take your patients seriously from now on and I hope that when another patient consults you in the future, you seriously reconsider your advice. The patient also has to consciously carry the risk of uncertainty or further examinations that will have to be carried out, until a 100 percent certainty is established."

More silence ensued before he apologised with the words: "I understand what you're telling me. I really am very, very sorry."

So I finally got closure and felt liberated!

- *Consulting a psycho-oncologist:* if one has the feeling of needing help for one's *mental wellbeing,* when one's own strength and the support from relatives and friends is not (or no longer) enough, in order to aid targeted therapeutic treatment in the healing process.
- *Living as normal a life as possible.* My grandmother considered work to be the best way to combat emotional pain. I tend to agree with her. Work helps in re-establishing a normal life. It is, however, important not to fall back into the same old rut and to ensure having a healthy diet, exercise and to live in a stress-free environment.

Although I am a psychologist, I am convinced that cancer can't be cured through positive thinking alone, but a healthy psyche does play an essential part, as one of the jigsaw puzzle pieces in the recovery process.

Physical activity and the immune system

As part of the immune system, the white blood cells in our body, also called *leucocytes*, serve to ward off infections. Most white blood cells are found in the bone marrow where they are being produced. Only a small percentage of them are in the blood. In the case of infections, but also during exercise, the leucocytes' activity increases and they search the entire organism for pathogens. They utilise the bloodstream to get from one site to the next while systematically scanning the walls of the vascular cells and trying to locate injuries and inflammations, as well as foreign predators such as cancer cells. White blood cells include T- lymphocytes which are particularly important for immune defence and tumour resistance. They are produced in the thymus gland which is located in the chest right behind the sternum. I've therefore made it a habit to activate this gland repeatedly by tapping it for a minute with the tips of my fingers or gently with my fist, just like Tarzan. Exercise and sport also stimulates excretions, detoxification through perspiring and blood flow to the tissue through increased oxygen supply. Moreover, physical exercise uses up larger amounts of glucose whereby the glucose stores are depleted and the blood sugar level remains low.

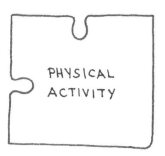

PHYSICAL ACTIVITY

Permitting that one's physical condition is acceptable, then moderate endurance training is advisable. Gerhard Uhlenbruck, an immunologist at the University of Cologne, reports an interesting connection between endurance training and training of the immune system. Exercising the muscles and the adjoining tissue triggers inflammation-like processes which, in turn, release messenger substances that stimulate the immune system. Thus immune cells acquire a certain aptitude in recognising foreign structures such as tumour cells. Even when cancer has already developed, sports activities can help to kick-start the immune system and aid the healing process. But be careful: the positive effects of exercising are reversed when training is excessive and the personal performance limit is constantly challenged. Peak performances and intensive exercise weaken the immune defence.

Ideally, one should aim for moderate endurance and strength training, with increased but relaxed breathing – relaxed enough to still be able to talk comfortably. This should generally correspond to a heart rate of 180 a minute minus a 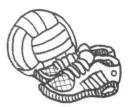 person's age, but always individually adjusted to that person's fitness level. One should exercise for at least half an hour a day. Suitable are swimming, walking, jogging and cycling, everything one enjoys or that the doctor recommends.

The right diet and sufficient outdoor exercise are important to stay healthy or regain one's health after a disease. However, it is just as important to get enough sleep.

Without sufficient sleep the body's regenerative capacity decreases and the immune system is weakened, one can get ill more easily and the risk of developing cancer significantly increases. In a study published in 2003, the psychiatrist David Spiegel and his colleague Sandra Sephton concluded that the hormone balance caused by sleep can help cancer patients in their fight against tumours. Here the cycle of being awake and sleeping acts on the metabolism through the hormones melatonin and cortisol. Melatonin, which the brain produces during sleep, has an antioxidative effect on harmful molecules, the free radicals. Furthermore melatonin also slows down oestrogen production in women. Without this natural deterrent too much oestrogen is produced which facilitates the development of hormone induced cancer types, such as ovarian and breast cancer. While we sleep at night, the body carries out intensive repairs on defective cell structures and DNA strands. For this reason it is important to ensure one gets enough and undisturbed sleep.

When the natural rhythm between sleeping and being awake is disrupted, the body's ability to regenerate itself and repair cell defects decreases, thus favouring the development of cancer. This was also shown in the evalution of numerous studies by the International Agency for Research on Cancer (IARC) of the World Health Organization (WHO), according to which people who work irregular night shifts are more prone to developing cancer. Irregular sleeping patterns evidently considerably weaken the immune system.

As the hormone melatonin, which is needed for a restful sleep, is only produced in darkness, I sleep in a darkened room. I also avoid stimulating drinks and food containing carbohydrates, as well as trying to avoid excitement or tension in order to lower my cortisol level, thereby making an enjoyable rest possible.

To calm down before going to bed, I try not to be "seduced" by television or the computer late at night.

I got all these tips from my grandmother. Since I've been following them, my body thanks me with wellbeing.

How I dealt with the side effects

In Japan, before the start of my radiotherapy, I had a consultation with one of the attending physicians who, amongst other things, explained possible side effects of the irradiation to me. At the time I wasn't overly interested in the subject. Following intensive research, I had decided on radiotherapy with carbon ions and wanted the treatment to start as quickly as possible. I would therefore have willingly signed any document to confirm that I was aware of potential side effects.

Today, however, I repeatedly take a look at the overview of side effects I'd been handed at the time. It's a valuable guideline to identifying possible future problems.

As is generally known carbon ion therapy and proton therapy are among the radiotherapies with the least side effects, whilst having a maximum effect on malignant tumours.

Yet short- as well as long-term side effects can occur.

Side effects I
personally experienced

I had hardly any short-term side effects. As already mentioned on page 79 et seq., thanks to cooling and treating my irradiated skin with olive oil, it saw very little damage. Drinking 3.5 litres of water and tea a day luckily also spared me from feeling nausea which frequently occurs as a consequence of poisoning symptoms.

Unfortunately, however, a year and a half after the radiotherapy I developed a massive side effect. But I will come to that later.

The first year after the treatment I felt extraordinarily well. Although the Japanese doctors believed that the nerves in the right side of my face wouldn't recover and this side of my face would subsequently remain paralysed, my facial nerves started functioning again a few months later. I'm extremely happy about the regeneration, that I'm practically no longer limited in my day to day life and that, at a first glance, nobody would suspect the terrible disease I had.

Today I enjoy looking into the mirror again and find myself quite attractive. It's a miracle, but a miracle that only materialised because I did everything in my power to help it along and always believed in it.

After that year, however, I suddenly felt inexplicable pains in my shoulder together with a rapid, one-sided muscular dystrophy in the throat, shoulder and back region. The pain became so intense that I had to carry my arm in a sling whenever I went on long walks. The muscles around the shoulder blade degenerated, my shoulder was no longer supported and slumped forward.

All the orthopaedists I visited, unanimously diagnosed an impingement syndrome (a functional impairment of the shoulder joint) and advised butterfly exercises to rebuild my muscles. But I didn't regard this as expedient seeing that I'd neither adopted a relieving posture nor been involved in an accident to justify the sudden abrupt muscular dystrophy. The recommended exercises wouldn't have been beneficial to my unilaterally weakened muscles but only further strengthened my already strong muscles and enhanced the asymmetry of my shoulder muscles.

The negative highlight of my consultation with those orthopaedists was one of their member's absurd assertion: "Men don't look at asymmetries in the neck and shoulder area." I was baffled. This was already the second time that I'd been given "advice" like that since I had started searching for medical help. My objection that I had consulted him because of my pain and not my appeal to the opposite sex, he dismissed with the instructions to his assistant that she should record my case as "impingement syndrome".

For the time being I could therefore not do anything but to keep moving and wait. Four months later I suddenly had extremely strong pains in my neck muscles and sometimes didn't know how to hold my head. I even took painkillers although I usually avoid them at all costs.

The pain subsided a few days later and I could also move my arm again. But naturally my muscle strength still hadn't been restored. Two months after this I also experienced headaches and nausea. This was always particularly bad at the start of the day and only marginally eased with some movement over the course of the morning.

I still didn't have any idea where these complaints stemmed from. My neck muscles kept deteriorating, my back hurt and I found it difficult to keep my head straight. For the summer holidays I bought a small air mattress to find some cooling relief when floating on it like a sack of potatoes in the water.

After the nausea and the weakening of my muscles became more and more unbearable, I decided to have a special MRI scan, a perfusion analysis, carried out in a hospital equipped to perform this type of examination. This way

I hoped to fully rule out the possibility that a new tumour could be causing the pain; my last MRI scan had revealed a small shadow which I had, however, more or less disregarded at the time. In retrospect, the *perfusion MRI*, which should differentiate between a tumour and necrosis (tissue damage), was diagnostically inconclusive as the bright shadow showed it was too close to the cranial bone. Therefore the perfusion MRI had to be evaluated just like a normal MRI, but I didn't know that at the time.

My mother and I tensely waited for the results; whilst waiting we decided to stay calm, in clear mind and not to be scared. Then I was handed the desired report. I opened it and started to read. They reported that there should exist three different tumours in my head.

My reaction was: "That's complete rubbish!"

But my mother fell apart although we had agreed to stay strong. She suddenly felt as if the carpet was being pulled from under her feet. Had she not be sitting down, she would have collapsed. She was completely and utterly shocked by the diagnosis: three tumours!

During the subsequent consultation, the doctor wanted to admit me as an inpatient right away and discuss the treatment planning approach and options with her colleagues. She explained the envisaged procedure and that brain surgery would probably be required for further clarification.

I thanked her, but declined for the time being. To counteract my dizziness and pain, it was suggested I could try taking cortisone. After checking my reflexes and on my request, another department issued me with a prescription for a week's supply of the hormone, which I immediately picked up on the way to my radiologist, who I very much trust. After assessing my head scan images, he suspected necrosis and a concomitant oedema (fluid accumulation). He based his assumption on my medical history and the fact that I actually seemed relatively perky to him, despite my severe headache. Then he kindly fetched me a glass of water so I could swallow the cortisone. While we discussed the images, my headache simply vanished. For weeks I had been struggling with dizziness, nausea and headaches and this was the first time I could properly breathe again. The feeling was so liberating, it literally removed a massive pressure. Although I'd received a terrible diagnosis just a few hours previously, I felt great!

I would like to point out that it can be life-saving to always have the images of a disease's progression evaluated by the same, competent radiologist. Being aware of the patient's medical history is extremely important when interpreting the images in order to avoid a misdiagnosis and therefore the wrong treatment. For the second time, my radiologist's expertise and diligence had provided me with the important foundation on which to base a medically correct decision.

Defining radiation necrosis

Radiation necrosis is tissue damage caused by radiotherapy. Necrosis, particularly when present in the brain, rates among the most severe complications associated with radiotherapy. Radiation necrosis mostly generates oedemas (water accumulation) which are especially dangerous in the head as they cause the intracranial pressure to increase. In my case this first became noticeable through muscle dystrophy in the shoulder and through nausea some months later. Treating necrosis in the brain is difficult, protracted and uncertain. Radiation necrosis is rare (five percent) and on average presents 14 months after radiotherapy. It is difficult to differentiate it from a recurring tumour because it occurs in the same area and looks similar on MR images.

I now had two choices:

- to have radiation necrosis surgically removed, which could, however, have led to dangerous complications as necrosis presents in the irradiated area and irradiated tissue has a very poor healing tendency, or
- to take cortisone over a prolonged period and hope that radiation necrosis in the brain would at some stage come to a halt and with it the oedema.

If not treated, radiation necrosis progresses and becomes irreversible. Radiation necrosis' growth and the associated oedema production, particularly in the brain, can prove to be fatal and lethal for the patient. This is even more dangerous in the case of younger patients because they still have a larger brain volume and the intracranial pressure therefore increases significantly faster. Diagnosing radiation necrosis in time can be life-saving.

I decided on the second of my options and took cortisone from then one. Cortisone is a hormone with a dampening effect on excessive reactions of the immune system and inhibits inflammation. Through taking it I endeavoured to keep necrosis and the associated oedema in check. In the first week I started with 8 mg of dexamethasone per day, reduced it to 4 mg per day in the second week and then took 3 mg per day over the following ones. During the course of a year I eventually lowered my intake to 1 mg a day.

In April 2013, however, despite regular cortisone intake on the preceding days, I woke up with a severe headache and extreme nausea. Subsequently I increased the cortisone dose over the following hours, but this was to no avail and I proceeded to vomit.

Hour by hour I became increasingly weaker until I could no longer stand or talk and briefly fainted. My mother and my partner called an ambulance which carried me away on a stretcher with the intention of delivering me to the stroke hospital.

But my mother was convinced that my condition had been caused by an increase of the brain oedema, presumably triggered by eating food that was too spicy. Thus I ended up in the neurosurgical ward. Here they insisted on taking a new CT scan before treating me although I had brought my current MR images with me on which the oedema was clearly visible. Unfortunately I had to wait three hours for this CT scan – feeling enormous pressure in my head and drugged up to my eyeballs with painkillers. In the end I was administered a high dose of cortisone by infusion and on my mother's insistence also a mannitol infusion (sugar alcohol which promotes fluid excretion from the body). A few hours later I felt better and the nightmare was finally over. Because the doctors at the hospital were convinced that necrosis was the cause of my condition and also believed it may have possibly triggered an epileptic-seizure, they prescribed an anti-epileptic drug. I didn't take it and never had another "attack" after that.

Pretty much a year later, however, I suffered from extreme nausea although I regularly took cortisone. This time we went to the hospital sooner where, on my express wish, I was given nothing but a mannitol infusion which I had even brought to the hospital myself. After my "seizure" the year before, I had provided myself with the infusion solution and ever since carried a bottle of it with me on all my trips in case of an emergency. Months before I had carefully read the instruction leaflet that came with my Mannitol 15% infusion bottle and therefore knew that, taking my body weight into account, two thirds of my 250 ml infusion bottle had to be administered inside 30 minutes. It is generally advisable to only have a mannitol infusion in emergencies as multiple applications can endanger the blood-brain barrier and also cause kidney damage.

The mannitol quickly extracted the water from my brain

and the huge pressure in my head rapidly subsided. Soon I felt better again. Not much later I was able to leave the ward unassisted, while only an hour and a half before I couldn't walk and had to be pushed in a wheelchair.

I was extremely happy that I didn't need a cortisone infusion this time, as the high cortisone doses had quite upset my stomach and I already had to fight major reflux symptoms, caused by prolonged cortisone intake.

It's also important to realise that cortisone preparations differ greatly in the quantity of active ingredients they contain. 1 mg of dexamethasone corresponds to roughly 25 mg of cortisol. Thus 0.75 mg of dexamethasone is more or less equivalent to the daily dose of the normal endogenous production.

Knowing this is incredibly important because it explains how, after a year of taking cortisone, it still took another year to reduce my dexamethasone intake from 1 mg to 0 mg. The body needs sufficient time to stimulate its own cortisol production again. Weaning oneself off too quickly, can be life-threatening.

It also has to be mentioned that cortisol lowers the DHEA hormone in the blood which can lead to fatigue and list-

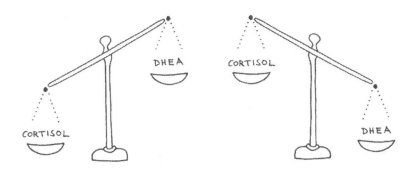

Fig. 23: When the DHEA level rises, the cortisol level drops. When the cortisol level rises, the DHEA level drops.

196

lessness. I therefore tried taking DHEA to counteract this. For me, however, this resulted in more severe headaches. Looking back it becomes clear that DHEA acted as an opponent to the cortisone I had taken and thus reduced its effect whereby the oedema production increased.

As I had also tried a *hyperbaric oxygen therapy* in my fight against radiation necrosis in the brain, I shall describe it here.

In hyperbaric oxygen therapy one breathes in pure oxygen through a mask in a compression chamber with increased ambient pressure (2.0 to 3.0 bar). Let me illustrate this. When diving into the ocean one reaches an ambient pressure of 2 bar at a depth of approx. 10 metres. The normal atmospheric ambient pressure at sea level, on the other hand, is circa 1 bar. The aim of hyperbaric oxygen therapy is to increase the oxygen content in the blood, as this can promote healing in cases such as:

- *emergencies* through smoke or carbon monoxide poisoning,
- *acute illnesses* like severe soft tissue injuries, compound fractures, burn wounds and
- *chronic* conditions such as badly healing wounds, radiotherapy side effects and many more.

Because hyperbaric oxygen therapy is also used to combat long term side-effects of radiotherapy such as necrosis, I completed several of these treatments.

In my case (radiation necrosis in the brain) though, I felt that necrosis was stimulated by the therapy, produced even more fluid and subsequently the pressure on my brain and my headaches increased. Although this may have been attributable to my necrosis trying to heal, based on this experience I can only recommend hyperbaric oxygen therapy for radiation necrosis in the brain with caution.

After finishing the therapy I had to take cortisone for another year until my necrosis had once and for all "calmed down" and stopped producing water! Two years after taking cortisone I was finally rewarded with success: my necrosis was arrested! It may have been risky, but patience and perseverance had more than paid off for me.

Heartburn – two years of cortisone intake affects the stomach

The side effects I'm about to outline were not primarily attributable to radiotherapy but to the cortisone intake it necessitated in my case.

1 mg of dexamethasone – the cortisone I had to take for two years because of its ability to pass the blood-brain barrier – corresponds to circa 25 mg of cortisol. This is slightly higher than the body's own daily production. I had to take on average 3 mg of dexamethasone per day for a year and on average 0.75 mg daily the following year; this illustrates the large amounts of cortisone I ingested. This first affected my stomach and later on also my joints. I tried a whole range of products to protect my stomach while taking cortisone, but they all caused massive side effects, so that I had to back away from them.

As early as a year after taking cortisone on a daily basis, I noticed that I suffered from recurrent bouts of heartburn. One and a half years later this became almost a daily occurrence. It manifested in a sore throat, especially right after swallowing the cortisone tablet. Even though I was able to reduce my cortisone intake over time, my stomach was more and more affected by it and reacted increasingly more sensitively to the daily dose. As I had absolutely no experience with heartburn, I consulted a specialist for reflux diseases, hoping that he could provide some dietary advice as well as telling me how to deal with heartburn. After listening to the account of my symptoms he diagnosed them as severe reflux. By now I had a sore throat every day and had to cough nearly every time I ate something, because my throat felt raw. As soon as I lay down, the coughing would start as well because acidic vapours would rise from the stomach and provoke an irritation of the throat, a so-called silent reflux.

Apart from the specialist's assertion that cortisone causes mood swings and depression, he only handed me a lot of further referrals including one for a mammography. My argument that I felt mentally well-adjusted and that I'd only just had a PET scan, which had in no way indicated any anomalies in my chest he ignored by saying, "That's exactly what I meant when I talked about mood swings!" Neither did he help me in any way as he was only prepared to provide nutritional advice after performing a gastroscopy during which some tissue samples for further analysis would be extracted. Because I didn't believe that anything malignant had developed in my oesophagus or stomach, I decided against a gastroscopy as my throat was already raw, my skin was thin and all my wounds healed very badly due to the cortisone. In the evening I surprisingly received a call from an anaesthetist unknown to me, who wanted to negotiate an appointment for a preliminary examination for the gastroscopy. He explained that I could come and see him at any time to discuss possible fears I had about the procedure. He also told me that I could call on him even if I decided not to go ahead with the gastroscopy. I secretly wondered why?

The incredible speed with which my phone number, which I had entrusted to the reflux specialist, was apparently circulated left me speechless.

By now I was determined that my stomach would have to endure until I could stop taking cortisone, in order to counteract necrosis and the oedema it induced. Thus I repeatedly tried to reduce my cortisone intake and succeeded.

I gradually lost the one and a half stone that I had gained

through taking cortisone. This was achieved by reducing the dosage to less than 1.5 mg of dexamethasone below the Cushing threshold. The Cushing threshold refers to the cortisone dose from where on the patient develops typical symptoms like moon face, thin, fragile skin or truncal obesity. The many months of cortisone intake above this Cushing threshold had in my case become most noticeably when my face started to bloat. But because of the reflux I didn't eat as much as before and my last meal before going to bed was at five in the afternoon. The proton pump inhibitors I had been prescribed (to protect the stomach) only caused side effects such as trembling, which was so severe that I wasn't even able to write anymore. Unfortunately although I tried many different products in varying dosages they sadly brought little relief. Only a dose of 10 mg of a certain proton pump inhibitor over four weeks in combination with a strict diet was physically manageable. All my stomach could handle was salads, fish or meat with as little fat as possible and a few potatoes now and then. Sweets and any kind of sugar instantly caused irritation in my throat, which was then followed by violent sneezing. After four weeks of 10mg of proton pump inhibitor I had to stop taking it, as it started to cause a rash.

When asked what types of food agreed with me, I replied: "Basically nothing!" Any kind of fruit, sweets and hot and spicy dishes were absolutely out of the question! Other dishes such as sushi without soya sauce, miso soup or Korean noodle soup, however, I could occasionally tolerate quite well. Cooked vegetables, oven chips with ketchup, potato chips with salt, but without flavour enhancers and yeast as well as rice with cheese or ham every so often, interestingly enough, agreed with me over a prolonged period and helped to keep the worst hunger pangs at bay. Milk and milk products gave me heartburn, although at the outset of the reflux disease a matcha latte had a soothing effect on my stomach. Some teas I tried also brought some relief for a certain amount of time, until I had to change the type of tea as my body had apparently become too accustomed to it and needed variety every now and then. Yarrow and wild mallow leaves tea were my favourites at that time, but sage tea and tea made from liquorice root also worked miracles for a while. Wheat bread, particularly when made with high performance wheat, disappeared from my diet altogether. Instead I could occasionally eat a slice of spelt bread, but only with butter or a spread so that the crumbs wouldn't immediately make me cough. Another "trick" was to eat quickly to ensure that at least some food ended up in my stomach before I had to cough. As soon as I started having to cough, I lost my appetite.

I thought it was also worth trying to line the stomach before taking cortisone, by eating linseed jelly for breakfast. This did actually help for a few days. Chestnut flour puree with liquorice root powder also featured on my breakfast menu for a while. It tasted quite good and provided some calories I badly needed at this stage as I was constantly losing weight.

Other remedies such as base powder or medicinal clay with zeolite brought no relief. They actually intensified the heartburn as the stomach's acid production was even more stimulated. I also tried Schüssler salt No. 9, which when I noticed that the acid in my stomach was getting out of control, I sometimes took one to two tablets of it, and this made it more bearable. Taken as a preventative or regular measure, however, made my condition deteriorate.

I guess everyone has to find out for themselves how to control heartburn. All I can do is give advice and describe what helped me.

After a year of reflux I weighed less than ever before in relation to my height and gradually started to worry about the weight loss. My trousers were flapping around my legs; my reserves would presumably be exhausted soon! But because I still had to take cortisone every day, which damaged my stomach lining even more, there was no escape from this vicious circle. "You have to be patient," my mother told me while enjoying some delicious chocolates. "It won't be long until you can stop the cortisone."

Dining out was no longer appealing, except at Japanese, Vietnamese or Korean restaurants which offered either sushi or noodle soups. Otherwise it was extremely difficult to find something suitable for me on the menu.

Almost two years later I was able to stop taking cortisone and dealt with the last remaining light headaches by having a cup of coffee in the morning. This was just in time as my stomach rejected nearly any kind of food I offered it. Now it would be revealed if I had been right to attribute my reflux to the cortisone I had been taking.

My stomach slowly healed and the severe cough when I was eating and during the night became less frequent. Soon I could also eat a few small pieces of fruit again. But I couldn't ask too much of my stomach yet because it would instantly retaliate with severe coughing fits. Whenever this happened, I had to keep to a strict diet for several days after.

Over the Christmas and New Year's Eve period I suffered an enormous setback. Desperately trying to gain another kilo, I had indulged in too much food, biscuits and wine and had to take 10 mg of proton pump inhibitors a day, for two days. But this time my stomach recovered relatively fast.

Even in those difficult "reflux periods" I repeatedly tried to support my stomach and immune system with alternative supplements. Amongst many others they included wild mallow leaves, yarrow and sage tea, the medicinal mushroom Hericium and L-lysine for the stomach lining, vitamin D and occasionally curcumin, which, although slightly spicy, is simply healthy and so important for the stomach and the intestines. Depending on my condition, I could sometimes take more and sometimes less of these.

Today I can clearly state that my stomach won and asserted itself against the cortisone. By now I can nearly eat everything again and occasionally even some delicious chocolate…

Other parts of my body, however, are still fighting the side effects of the two year long cortisone therapy.

Joint pains – a side effect of taking cortisone

When my joint pains became so severe that they woke me up during the night, I made an appointment at a hospital's rheumatism outpatient department. As I couldn't get an appointment for two weeks later, I had to think of an interim solution and started researching dietary supplements to combat joint pains, which I was then able to procure that same day.

Soon after, the pain luckily became more bearable, which I attributed to taking those dietary supplements.

I still kept my appointment at the rheumatism outpatient department where they merely suggested cortisone infusion treatment. Since I was convinced that my joint pains had been caused by my prolonged cortisone intake, this was out of the question.

So it was entirely up to me to relieve the pain. These were my basic considerations:

Long-term cortisone intake adversely influences the calcium metabolism (see the dexamethasone instruction leaflet) and facilitates osteoperosis and atrophy of the muscles which has to be counteracted in time. It is therefore important to supply the body with sufficient amounts of calcium and vitamin D while taking cortisone. Which I did, yet I wasn't able to prevent extreme muscle and joint pains.

So what else could I take to come to grips with the pain in the short and long term?

My mother advised me to be patient. She was convinced that these pains would also subside over time, the same way my stomach pains had. But I wanted to speed up the pain relief, seeing that I suffered every day. During the course of our further research we eventually discovered additional natural remedies. Taking these for several months significantly improved my condition.

My "remedies" for joint pains

The following remedies all support healthy physiological processes, build up the whole body and are anti-inflammatory thereby reducing pain while simultaneously preventing cancer.

MSM – organic sulphur

MSM (abbreviation of methylsulfonylmethane) is an organic sulphur compound which can favourably influence many metabolic processes in the body. Sulphur is an essential component of vital amino acids like *cysteine* or *methionine*.

On the one hand they have vital functions for the metabolism, on the other they are required in the production of proteins which are the basic building blocks of all human cells.

Sulphur is an important component of glutathione which significantly contributes to the body's own immune defence as well as the fight against free radicals. As a constituent part of glutathione peroxidase, glutathione counteracts the consequences of oxidative stress. In the fight against cancer an increase of the glutathione level has also shown positive effects.

As the proportion of sulphur in our diet has been reduced through changed environmental conditions in agriculture, this can lead to a deficiency of this important mineral which can be counterbalanced through dietary supplements such as MSM.

Successful results through MSM intake have, among others, been recorded in the case of arthrosis pain, osteoporosis, various allergies and heartburn. I noticed the positive influence of MSM in particular in the alleviation of the joint pains that had been caused by my prolonged cortisone intake. Sulphur is contained in the joint lubricants and the inner layer of joint capsules. The body has to continuously renew both of these for which it requires sulphur. When sulphur is missing, painful signs of degeneration and stiff joints are the result. Arthritically damaged cartilage contains roughly two thirds less sulphur than healthy cartilage. MSM can therefore also protect against joint inflammation and cartilage degradation. As thermal water usually also contains sulphur it contributes towards relieving joint pains.

MSM is one of my favourite dietary supplements and I take it regularly in capsule form. As already mentioned, it helps alleviate my joint pains, is anticarcinogenic and also agrees with my stomach due to its acid regulating function.

Krill oil

In one of the previous chapters I have already described its significance, however, I only took larger quantities once I needed to relieve my joint pains. Krill oil as an important omega 3 fatty acid supplier, plays a special role in counteracting omega 6 and omega 9 fatty acids and therefore an essential one in the protection against inflammations. Its effectiveness shows in the blood count, with the aid of the CRP value (an inflammation parameter) for instance, which can be lowered by taking krill oil. The immediately absorbable phospholipids contained in krill oil are helpful in the body's overall regeneration and have an important role in delaying cartilage degradation. Moreover, krill oil also reduces deposits in the vessels and is mood-enhancing.

Capsules to aid joint and cartilage repair

To aid joint and cartilage repair, I also take capsules consisting of natural substances such as glucosamine sulphate and chondroitin sulphate as well as coral limestone. Glucosamine is an amino sugar and a component of connective tissue, cartilage and synovial fluid. Chondroitin sulphate is an important building block of cartilage tissue and ensures its pressure resistance. Together they work synergistically and have a cartilage protecting and possibly cartilage repairing effect.

I have the impression that taking these remedies also positively affected my joints.

Astaxanthin

Astaxanthin is a carotenoid and an especially powerful antioxidant which can be found in certain algae. When animals like salmon, lobster, shrimps, crabs or flamingos eat large amounts of these algae, they accumulate astaxanthin in their bodies, especially the muscles, and turn pink.

Astaxanthin prevents the oxidation processes of free radicals and is anti-inflammatory. Moreover, astaxanthin has the ability to overcome the blood-brain barrier and so protects the brain and the nerves from free radicals and inflammations. It can also surmount the blood-retinal barrier, thus frequently taking astaxanthin improves eyesight.

Astaxanthin therefore counteracts numerous diseases which are caused by chronic inflammations. Amongst others, these include arthritis and Crohn's disease. According to a study the intake of high doses of astaxanthin (40 mg per day) also reduces reflux complaints. As low inflammation parameters in the blood can also impede the probability of cancer recurrence, I take astaxanthin capsules.

Does the chance of recovery increase when several conventional treatment options are promptly employed?

The answer to this question is tricky. My deliberations are as follows: All conventional treatments, especially chemotherapy, extensive surgery or radiotherapy, severely weaken the endogenous immune system. This makes it difficult for the body to fight possibly remaining cancer cells on its own after several orthodox treatments. I believed that in my case the suggested surgery, estimated to take about 18 hours, followed by conventional radiotherapy, would overtax my resources. For that reason, amongst others, I decided on "just" radiotherapy, but a highly precise and efficient form of it. Some patients with the same disease as mine made a different decision. After surgery they had extensive, conventional irradiation "to be on the safe side" although their tumours had been entirely removed following recommendations by their physicians. However, should a relapse occur in the irradiated area, repeat radiation treatment is no longer possible or extremely risky due to the expected side effects (e.g. uncontrollable, life-threatening necrosis). Operating on the irradiated area again is also problematic in view of the tissue's decreased tendency to heal.

As for my type of tumour (ACC) chemotherapy is virtually non-effective and conventional immunotherapy is not proven to be effective, patients with the disease are quickly considered to be incurable. Very often people hastily say it should be irradiated, just to be on the safe side. This therefore forfeits an important future option.

Based on my personal experience, I recommend: as much conventional treatment as necessary, but, at the same time, as little conventional treatment as possible.

The following page shows a "schedule" outlining the ten most important stages from diagnosis to cure.

Recovery schedule

Get diagnosed and stay calm.

Educate yourself about the cancer type's characteristics and growth pattern – become an expert in the field yourself.

Gather information regarding the treatment options from several medical professionals and through your own research.

Contact different clinics for treatment

Send your medical reports to various renowned clinics and enquire how and with what chances of success they would treat the disease. Should you consider treatment abroad, ask about the costs.

In the case of a justified wish to get treated abroad, send a request to cover the costs to your health insurance provider.

Decide on the treatment – only after diligent deliberation, using your common sense.

This should be done together with a trusted doctor and maybe family and/or friends. If possible keep your options for additional future treatments open.

Have the treatment – a very significant step towards recovery.

Build-up your immune system.

After having conventional treatment it is important to strengthen the immune system through a healthy diet, selected dietary supplements, moderate exercise, living in a healthy environment and maintaining psychological wellbeing.

Have regular check-ups to provide clarity and security.

Cure: After five cancer-free years one can talk of cure.

Conclusion

"Cure" is an incredibly strong word. Every patient should include it in his vocabulary and make it his goal.

With the right choice of treatment and an intelligent, life-long, balanced diet, psychological wellbeing and exercise in healthy surroundings, one has an excellent chance of regaining the control over one's body and to be cured from cancer. Should other complaints occur at a later stage, however, one should always consider the original cancer in one's deliberations.

Long-term consequences, even those as severe as my radiation necrosis in the brain, are usually very treatable, provided they are diagnosed in time. I explored my own disease in great detail, put myself in charge of it, carefully selected the correct treatment for me from numerous options and didn't just leave the responsibility with the specialists.

No doubt, my cancer changed my life, I was made aware of its finite nature at a young age. Therefore I now live more consciously, enjoy nature's beauty and uniqueness possibly more intensively than most others, and consider each day I live to be a gift. Today I can live a normal life and it is no longer apparent that I once suffered from a severe disease. My dream of regaining my facial functions and quality of life has come true, despite the experts' statements to the contrary.

For the future, I wish that conventional medicine and naturopathy work hand in hand to heal the patient. Both specialist fields should be synergistically employed for the patient's benefit. Everyone should take their road to recovery into their own hands. With this book I hope to have provided some substantial support according to the motto:

Ask everybody, take what you need and leave the rest!

Acknowledgements

Very special thanks go to my husband Georg and to my mother Sonja. With their unconditional love and backing they not only supported me on the road to recovery, but also in the process of writing this book.

A special thank you is also due to my radiologist Dr Erich Steiner, Clinical Senior Lecturer. His timely, correct interpretation of my scans greatly contributed to my recovery. He also motivated me to write this book to help other patients to take personal responsibility for their disease, but also to provide doctors with an insight into a patient's psyche.

A big thank to the fantastic team in Japan. Their innovative treatment saved my life in a way worth living.

I am also grateful to the medical professionals among my circle of friends and to my native speaking friends, for their constructive feedback regarding the content and the translation of this book.

Last, but not least, a heartfelt thank you to my friend Maria-Michaela V. Borejko, who graphically implemented my optical concepts with her illustrations.

References

Prologue

WHO (2013): Latest World Cancer Statistics. Press Release 223, 12. 12. 2013, www.iarc.fr/en/media-centre/pr/2013/pdfs/pr223_E.pdf, (last accessed September 2017).

Exploring conventional medical options

Birkenmeier, A. (2014): Immuntherapie bei Krebs. www.unispital-basel.ch/fileadmin/unispitalbaselch/Medien/Medienspiegel/20140201_medienspiegel_mediaplanet_krebs.pdf, (last accessed September 2017).
Creutzig, U. & Klusmann, J.-H. (2002): Von tödlichen zu heilbaren Krankheiten. Die Erfolge der Pädiatrischen Onkologie in den letzten 25 Jahren. Gesellschaft für pädiatrische Onkologie und Hämatologie, 22. 11. 2002, www.kinderkrebsinfo.de/sites/kinderkrebsinfo/content/e1812/e1946/e1936/e88507/ErfolgsgeschichtePOH_2002-12_ger.pdf, (last accessed September 2017).
http://derstandard.at/2000014325600/Immuntherapie-soll-Krebsbehandlung-verbessern, 15. 4. 2015, (last accessed September 2017).
http://global.onclive.com/web-exclusives/the-role-of-anti-pd-l1-immunotherapy-in-cancer, 29. 1. 2014, (last accessed September 2017).

http://symptomat.de/Antikörpertherapie, (last accessed September 2017).

Losch, F.O. (2001): Aktivierung von T-Lymphozyten durch melanomspezifische variante Antigen-Rezeptoren. Dissertation. Albert-Ludwigs-Universität Freiburg.

Lønning, P.E. (2011): The potency and clinical efficacy of aromatase inhibitors across the breast cancer continuum. Ann Oncol, 22(3): pp. 503–514. doi: 10.1093/annonc/mdq337

Mauritz, E. (2014): Immuntherapien gegen Krebs: „Aufregend und verblüffend". kurier.at, 2. 7. 2014, http://kurier.at/wissen/neue-immuntherapien-als-hoffnung-im-kampf-gegen-krebs/72.907.869, (last accessed September 2017).

Mauritz, E. (2015a): Immuntherapie ist wirksamer als Chemotherapie. kurier.at, 15. 4. 2015, http://kurier.at/lebensart/gesundheit/immuntherapie-ist-wirksamer-als-chemotherapie/125.304.224, (last accessed September 2017).

Mauritz, E. (2015b): Neue Sicht auf Krebs: „Wie ein Organ". kurier.at, 14. 7. 2015, http://kurier.at/lebensart/gesundheit/neue-sicht-auf-krebs-wie-ein-organ/141.299.062, (last accessed September 2017).

Mittler, D. (2015): Wie der Körper Krebs selbst besiegen könnte. Sueddeutsche Zeitung online, 15. 7. 2015, www.sueddeutsche.de/bayern/forschung-revolutionaere-zellen-1.2566999, (last accessed September 2017).

Rody, A., Loibl, S., von Minckwitz, G. & Kaufmann, M. (2005): Use of goserelin in the treatment of breast cancer. Expert Rev Anticancer Ther, 5(4): pp. 5904. doi: 10.1586/14737140.5.4.591

Seiter, H. (Hrsg.), Aulitzky, W.E. (Hrsg.) & Waldmann, W. (Hrsg.) (2007): Handbuch Krebs: Alles zu Vorsorge, Diagnose, Therapiemöglichkeiten und Heilungschancen. Mit Arzt- und Klinikführer. München: Südwest Verlag.

Sommer, K. (2011): Krebstherapie: Was ist möglich? lifeline.de, 18. 1. 2011, www.lifeline.de/themenspecials/krebs/krebstherapie-was-ist-moeglich-id37423.html, (last accessed September 2017).

Stadler, J. (2015): Krebsmedizin. Derzeit glücken Forschern gewaltige Fortschritte bei der Therapie wie auch bei einem tieferen Verständnis der Tumorentstehung. profil wissen, Das Wissenschaftsmagazin der Profil-Redaktion, Nr. 1, 18. 03. 2015: pp. 14–29.

Stamatiadis-Smidt, H., zur Hausen, H., Wiestler, O.D. & Gebest, H.-J. (Hrsg.) (2006): Thema Krebs. 3. Aufl., Heidelberg: Springer Medizin Verlag.

Stenman, U.-H., Alfthan, H. & Hotakainen, K. (2004): Human chorionic gonadotropin in cancer. Clin Biochem, 37(7): pp. 549–61. doi: 10.1016/j.clinbiochem.2004.05.008

Witte, F. (2015): Schwanger trotz Krebs. derStandard.at, 7. 6. 2015, http://derstandard.at/2000016030276/Schwanger-trotz-Krebs, (last accessed September 2017).

www.cancer.ca/en/cancer-information/diagnosis-and-treatment/tests-and-procedures/human-chorionic-gonadotropin-hcg-or-b-hcg/, (last accessed September 2017).

www.onkologie.hexal.de/arzneimittel/hormontherapie/, (last accessed September 2017).

www.rptc.de/de/therapieablauf/kombinationstherapien/bestrahlung-plus-operation.html, (last accessed September 2017).

Akamatsu, H., Karasawa, K., Omatsu, T. et al. (2014): First experience of carbon-ion radiotherapy for early breast cancer. Jpn J Radiol, 32(5): pp. 288–295. doi: 10.1007/s11604–014–0300–6

Akino, Y., Teshima, T., Kihara, A. et al. (2009): Carbon-ion beam irradiation effectively suppresses migration and invasion of human non-small-cell lung cancer cells. Int J Radiat Oncol Biol Phys, 75(2): 475–481. doi: 10.1016/j.ijrobp.2008.12.090

Amaldi, U. & Kraft, G. (2005): Recent applications of Synchrotrons in cancer therapy with Carbon Ions. Europhysics News, Vol. 36(4): pp. 114–118. doi: 10.1051/epn:2005402

Combs, S.E., Schulz-Ertner, D., Herfarth, K.K. et al. (2006): Fortschritte in der Radioonkologie – Von der Präzisionsstrahlentherapie mit Photonen zur Ionentherapie mit Protonen und Kohlenstoffionen. Der Chirurg, 77(12): pp. 1126–1132. doi: 10.1007/s00104–006–1268–2

Ellerbrock, M. (2009): Strahlentherapie mit Protonen/Schwerionen. DEGRO-Jahreskongress, Bremen, 11.-14. 06. 2009, www.degro.org/dav/html/kongress2009/refresher/ellerbrock.pdf, (last accessed September 2017).

Europäisches Cyberknife Zentrum München-Großhadern (2012): Strahlenmesser schaltet Tumoren aus. Pressemitteilung, www.cyber-knife.net/fileadmin/user_upload/Pressemeldungen/Cyberknife-Forschungskooperation-12.pdf, (last accessed September 2017).

Hass, F. (2010): Jürgen Debus beschießt Tumore mit Schwerionen. berliner-zeitung.de, 17. 4. 2010, www. berliner-zeitung.de/archiv/juergen-debus-beschiesst-tumore-mit-schwerionen-krebsbehandlung-aus-dem-teilchenbeschleuniger---mit-protonen--und-schwerionenstrahlen-lassen-sich-tumore-wesentlich-exakter-und-effektiver-beschiessen-als-mit-herkoemmlichen-roentgenstrahlen--man-braucht-nur-ein-drittel-der-dosis-,10810590,10711442.html, (last accessed September 2017).

http://de.slideshare.net/fovak/heidelberg-ion-therapy-center, (last accessed September 2017).

http://flexikon.doccheck.com/de/Brachytherapie, (last accessed September 2017).

Karasawa, K., Fujita, M., Shoji, Y. et al. (2014): Biological Effectiveness of Carbon-Ion Radiation on Various Human Breast Cancer Cell Lines. J Cell Sci Ther, 5(5):180. doi: 10.4172/2157-7013.1000180

Kato, S., Ohno, T., Tsujii, H. et al. (2006): Dose escalation study of carbon ion radiotherapy for locally advanced carcinoma of the uterine cervix. Int J Radiat Oncol Biol Phys, 65(2): 388–397. doi: 10.1016/j.ijrobp.2005.12.050

Koto, M., Hasegawa, A., Takagi, R. et al. (2014): Carbon Ion Radiotherapy for Head and Neck Cancer. J Radiol Radiat Ther, 2(2):1044.

Langbein, K. (2012): Radieschen von oben. Über Leben mit Krebs. Salzburg: Ecowin Verlag.

Leiser, D., Malyapa, R., Schneider, R. & Weber, D. (2015): Die Protonentherapie – Anwendungsspektrum und Indikationen. Schweizer Zeitschrift für Onkologie, 01/2015: pp. 14–17.

Muacevic, A., Wowra, B. & Tonn, J.-C. (2007): Strahlenmesser lässt inoperable Tumoren verschwinden. MMW – Fortschritte der Medizin, 149(7): pp. 42–43.

Sauer, R. (2010): Strahlentherapie und Onkologie. 5. Aufl., München: Urban & Fischer Verlag.

Schulz-Ertner, D., Didinger, B., Nikoghosyan, A. et al. (2003): Optimization of radiation therapy for locally advanced adenoid cystic carcinomas with infiltration of the skull base using photon intensity-modulated radiation therapy (IMRT) and a carbon ion boost. Strahlenther Onkol, 179(5): 345–351. doi: 10.1007/s00066-003-1071-7

Stadler, J. (2015): Reportage. Ein Teilchenbeschleuniger im Süden Wiens soll die Krebstherapie revolutionieren. profil wissen, Das Wissenschaftsmagazin der Profil-Redaktion, Nr. 1, 18. 03. 2015: pp. 32–35.

Trautwein, A.X., Kreibig, U. & Hüttermann, J. (2008): Physik für Mediziner, Biologen, Pharmazeuten. 7. Aufl., Berlin: Walter de Gruyter GmbH und Co. KG.

Tsujii, H. & Kamada, T. (2012): A review of update clinical results of carbon ion radiotherapy. Jpn J Clin Oncol, 42(8): pp. 670–685. doi: 10.1093/jjco/hys104

Tsujii, H., Mizoe, J., Kamada, T. et al. (2007): Clinical Results of Carbon Ion Radiotherapy at NIRS. J Radiat Res, 48(Suppl A): A1– A13. doi: 10.1269/jrr.48.A1

van Weert, S., Reinhard, R., Bloemena, E. et al. (2016): Differences in patterns of survival in metastatic adenoid cystic carcinoma of the head and neck. Head Neck, 39(3): pp. 456–463. doi: 10.1002/hed.24613

Wannemacher, M., Debus, J. & Wenz, F. (Hrsg.) (2006): Strahlentherapie. Berlin, Heidelberg: Springer-Verlag.

www.dkfz.de/de/medphys/projekte/teilchentherapie.html, (last accessed September 2017).

www.gamma-knife.de/de/behandlung/behandlung.php, (last accessed September 2017).

www.gsi.de/forschungbeschleuniger/forschung_ein_ueberblick/ionenstrahlen_im_kampf_gegen_krebs/kohlenstoffionen_hochwirksam_und_praezise.htm (last accessed September 2017).

www.helmholtz.de/fileadmin/user_upload/05_aktuelles/ Termine_Veranstaltungen/helmholtz/Helmholtz_Salon/ Haberer_Ionenskalpell_Helmholtzsalon_public.pdf, (last accessed September 2017).

www.hirntumorhilfe.de/hirntumor/hirntumortherapie/ strahlentherapie/gammaknife, (last accessed September 2017).

www.klinikum.uni-heidelberg.de/Prof-Debus-Klinik.113189.0.html, (last accessed September 2017).

www.luks.ch/standorte/luzern/kliniken/radio-onkologie/ infrastruktur/linearbeschleuniger.html, (last accessed March 2016).

www.marienkrankenhaus.com/kliniken-institute/klinik-fuer-radio-onkologie/patienteninformation/was-bedeutet-afterloading, (last accessed September 2017).

www.medaustron.at/de/ionentherapie, (last accessed September 2017).

www.meduniwien.ac.at/hp/neurochirurgie/forschung/ wissenschaftliche-aktivitaeten/gamma-knife, (last accessed September 2017).

www.mh-hannover.de/strahlentherapie-hochpraezision. html, (last accessed September 2017).

www.onmeda.de/behandlung/strahlentherapie.html, (last accessed September 2017).

www.psi.ch/protontherapy/klinische-erfahrung, (last accessed September 2017).

www.ptcog.ch/index.php/facilities-in-operation, (last accessed September 2017).

www.rptc.de/de/protonentherapie/behandlungsspektrum. html, (last accessed September 2017).

www.rptc.de/de/therapieablauf/kombinationstherapien/ bestrahlung-plus-operation.html, (last accessed September 2017).

www.strahlentherapie.ukw.de/fuer-aerzte/ausstattung-und-techniken/bildgefuehrte-strahlentherapie-igrt.html, (last accessed September 2017).

www.strahlentherapie-sued.de/index.php?pg=intensitaetsmodulierte_strahlentherapie.php, (last accessed September 2017).

www.teilchen.at/kdm/17, (last accessed September 2017).

www.umweltinstitut.org/fileadmin/Mediapool/Downloads/01_Themen/01_Radioaktivitaet/umweltinstitut_strahlentherapie.pdf, (last accessed September 2017).

www.umweltinstitut.org/themen/radioaktivitaet/radioaktivitaet-und-gesundheit/medizin.html, (last accessed September 2017).

www.visionlearning.com/en/library/Chemistry/1/Atomictheory-II/51, (last accessed September 2017).

Inevitable certainty – torn between agony and hope

Akino, Y., Teshima, T., Kihara, A. et al. (2009): Carbon-ion beam irradiation effectively suppresses migration and invasion of human non-small-cell lung cancer cells. Int J Radiat Oncol Biol Phys, 75(2): pp. 475–481. doi: 10.1016/j.ijrobp.2008.12.090

Pommier, P., Liebsch, N.J., Deschler, D.G. et al. (2006): Proton beam radiation therapy for skull base adenoid cystic carcinoma. Arch Otolaryngol Head Neck Surg, 132(11): pp. 1242–1249. doi: 10.1001/archotol.132.11.1242

Schulz-Ertner, D., Didinger, B., Nikoghosyan, A. et al. (2003): Optimization of radiation therapy for locally advanced adenoid cystic carcinomas with infiltration of the skull base using photon intensity-modulated radiation therapy (IMRT) and a carbon ion boost. Strahlenther Onkol, 179(5): pp. 345-351. doi: 10.1007/s00066-003-1071-7

Schulz-Ertner, D., Nikoghosyan, A., Didinger, B. et al. (2005): Therapy strategies for locally advanced adenoid cystic carcinomas using modern radiation therapy techniques. Cancer, 104(2): pp. 338-344. doi: 10.1002/cncr.21158

Shimokawa, T., Ma, L., Ando, K. et al. (2016): The Future of Combining Carbon-Ion Radiotherapy with Immunotherapy: Evidence and Progress in Mouse Models. Int J Particle Ther, 3(1): pp. 61-70. doi: 10.14338/IJPT-15-00023.1

Tsujii, H. & Kamada, T. (2012): A review of update clinical results of carbon ion radiotherapy. Jpn J Clin Oncol, 42(8): pp. 670-685. doi: 10.1093/jjco/hys104

van Weert, S., Reinhard, R., Bloemena, E. et al. (2016): Differences in patterns of survival in metastatic adenoid cystic carcinoma of the head and neck. Head Neck, 39(3): pp. 456-463. doi: 10.1002/hed.24613

Wannemacher, M., Debus, J. & Wenz, F. (Hrsg.) (2006): Strahlentherapie. Berlin, Heidelberg: Springer-Verlag.

Hopeful journey to Japan

http://kurier.at/chronik/niederoesterreich/medaustron-vor-start-des-probebetriebs/35.727.505, (last accessed September 2017).

http://noe.orf.at/news/stories/2616431, (last accessed September 2017).

Kamada, T., Tsujii, H., Blakely, E.A. et al. (2015): Carbon ion radiotherapy in Japan: an assessment of 20 years of clinical experience Lancet Oncol, 16(2): e93-e100. doi: 10.1016/S1470-2045(14)70412-7

McLaughlin, N., Annabi, B., Lachambre, M.-P. et al. (2006): Combined low dose ionizing radiation and green tea-derived epigallocatechin-3-gallate treatment induces human brain endothelial cells death. J Neurooncol, 80(2): pp. 111-121. doi: 10.1007/s11060-006-9171-8

Reischl, G. (2015): Mit 200.000 Kilometer pro Sekunde gegen Krebszellen, futurezone.at, 16. 1. 2015, https://futurezone.at/science/mit-200-000-kilometer-pro-sekunde-gegen-krebszellen/108.323.180, (last accessed September 2017).

Stadler, J. (2015): Reportage. Ein Teilchenbeschleuniger im Süden Wiens soll die Krebstherapie revolutionieren. profil wissen, Das Wissenschaftsmagazin der Profil-Redaktion, Nr. 1, 18. 03. 2015, pp. 32–35.

www.medaustron.at, (last accessed September 2017).

After conventional therapy – personal responsibility continues

Bignold, L.P. (2006): Cancer: Cell Structures, Carcinogens and Genomic Instability. Basel: Birkhäuser Verlag.

Ferenčík, M., Rovenský, J., Maťha, V. & Herold, M. (2006): Kompendium der Immunologie: Grundlagen und Klinik. Wien: Springer-Verlag.

Folkman, J. (1991): Antiangiogenesis. In: Biologic Therapy of Cancer. DeVita, V.T., Hellman, S., Rosenberg, S.A. (Hrsg.), Philadelphia: J.B. Lippincott Company.

Ganten, D. & Ruckpaul, K. (Hrsg.) (2011): Herz-Kreislauf-Erkrankungen. Handbuch der Molekularen Medizin. Berlin: Springer Verlag.

Graw, J. (Hrsg.), Alberts, B., Bray, D., Hopkin, K. et al. (2012): Lehrbuch der Molekularen Zellbiologie. 4. Aufl., Weinheim: WILEY-VCH Verlag GmbH & Co. KGaA.

Hiddemann, W. (Hrsg.) & Bartram, C. (Hrsg.) (2010): Die Onkologie. Teil 1: Allgemeiner Teil: Epidemiologie – Pathogenese – Grundprinzipien der Therapie. Teil 2: Spezieller Teil: Solide Tumoren – Lymphome – Leukämien. 2. Aufl., Heidelberg: Springer Medizin Verlag.

Houghton, J., Stoicov, C., Nomura, S. et al. (2004): Gastric cancer originating from bone marrow-derived cells. Science, 306(5701): pp. 1568–1571. doi: 10.1126/science.1099513

http://flexikon.doccheck.com/de/Angiostatin, (last accessed September 2017).

Kröger, A. (2016): Immunsystem stabilisieren: Krebs VORBEUGEN und HEILEN! Kindle Edition.

Marx, J. (2004): Inflammation and cancer: The link grows stronger. Science. 306(5698): pp. 966–968. doi: 10.1126/science.306.5698.966

Ober, C., Sinatra, S. & Zucker, M. (2012): Earthing – Heilendes Erden: Gesund und voller Energie mit Erdkontakt. Kirchzarten: VAK Verlags GmbH.

O'Reilly, M.S., Holmgren, L., Shing, Y. et al. (1994): Angiostatin: a novel angiogenesis inhibitor that mediates the suppression of metastases by a Lewis lung carcinoma. Cell, 79(2): pp. 315–328.

Paetz, B. (2013): Chirurgie für Pflegeberufe. 22. Aufl., Stuttgart: Georg Thieme Verlag KG.

www.laborjournal.de/rubric/archiv/stichwort/w_98_02. lasso, (last accessed September 2017).

The importance of a proper diet and dietary supplements

Aggarwal, B.B., Kumar, A. & Bharti, A.C. (2003): Anticancer potential of curcumin: preclinical and clinical studies. Anticancer Res. 23(1A): pp. 363–398.

Amin, A.R.M., Zang H. & Shin, D.M. (2013): Molecular Aspects of Cancer Prevention by Green Tea: An overview. In: Tea in Health and Disease Prevention. pp. 751–766, London/Waltham/San Diego: Academic Press. doi: 10.1016/B978-0-12-384937-3.00063-X

Appendino, G., Belcaro, G., Cornelli, U. et al. (2010): Potential role of curcumin phytosome (Meriva) in controlling the evolution of diabetic microangiopathy. A pilot study. Panminerva Med, 53(3 Suppl 1): pp. 43–49.

Barry, R. (2011): Ubiquinol-Q10 – die Revolution in der Herztherapie. Kerkrade: Food for Health Publishing Media BV.

Beckmann, H. (2009): Die Anti-Krebs-Strategie: Krebs – und was man selbst dagegen tun kann! Norderstedt: Books on Demand GmbH.

Béliveau, R. & Gingras, D. (2010): Krebszellen mögen keine Himbeeren. Nahrungsmittel gegen Krebs. 6. Aufl., München: Wilhelm Goldmann Verlag.

Bertsche, T. & Schulz, M. (2003): Amygdalin – ein neues altes Krebsmittel? In: Pharmazeutische Zeitung online 24/2003, www.pharmazeutische-zeitung.de/index. php?id=pharm4_24_2003, (last accessed September 2017).

Beuth, J. & Drebing, V. (2006): Selen gegen Krebs: Unterstützung in der Tumorprävention und -therapie. Stuttgart: TRIAS Verlag.

Beuth, J. (2011): Gesund bleiben nach Krebs: Was Sie jetzt stärkt und schützt – Was hilft und einen Rückfall abwehrt. München: Wilhelm Goldmann Verlag.

Bhagavan, H.N. & Chopra, R.K. (2007): Plasma coenzyme Q10 response to oral ingestion of coenzyme Q10 formulations. Mitochondrion, 7 Suppl: pp. 78–88. doi: 10.1016/j.mito.2007.03.003

Budwig, J. (2013): Öl-Eiweiß-Kost. Kernen: Sensei Verlag.

Burke, D. (2009): Salvestrole – Neue Möglichkeiten der Krebsbehandlung. OM & Ernährung, Internationales Journal für orthomolekulare und verwandte Medizin. Nr. 129.

Cao, Y. & Cao, R. (1999): Angiogenesis inhibited by drinking tea. Nature 398: p. 381. doi: 10.1038/18793

Chang, H.-K., Shin, M.S., Yang, H.-Y. et al. (2006): Amygdalin induces apoptosis through regulation of Bax and Bcl-2 expressions in human DU145 and LNCaP prostate cancer cells. Biol Pharm Bull, 29(8): pp. 1597–1602.

Chatterjee, S.J., Ovadje, P., Mousa, M. et al. (2011): The efficacy of dandelion root extract in inducing apoptosis in drug-resistant human melanoma cells. Evid Based Complement Alternat Med, 2011:129045. doi: 10.1155/2011/129045

Chen, Y., Ma, J., Wang, F. et al. (2013): Amygdalin induces apoptosis in human cervical cancer cell line HeLa cells. Immunopharmacol Immunotoxicol, 35(1): pp. 43–51. doi: 10.3109/08923973.2012.738688

Clevers, H. (2011): The cancer stem cell: premises, promises and challenges. Nat Med, 17(3): pp. 313–319. doi: 10.1038/nm.2304

Cooke, M., Iosia, M., Buford, T. et al. (2008): Effects of acute and 14-day coenzyme Q10 supplementation on exercise performance in both trained and untrained individuals. J Int Soc Sports Nutr, 5:8. doi: 10.1186/1550-2783-5-8

Cordain, L., Eaton, S.B., Sebastian, A. et al. (2005): Origins and evolution of the Western diet: health implications for the 21st century. Am J Clin Nutr, 81(2): pp. 341–354.

Coy, J.F., Baumann, F.T., Spitz, J. & Cavelius, A. (2011): Die 8 Anti-Krebs-Regeln: Gesund im Einklang mit unseren steinzeitlichen Genen. München: Gräfe und Unzer Verlag GmbH.

Cunnane, S.C. (Hrsg.) & Thompson, L.U. (Hrsg.) (2003): Flaxseed in human nutrition. Second Edition. Champaign, Illinois: AOCS Press.

Curl, C.L., Fenske, R.A. & Elgethun, K. (2003): Organophosphorus pesticide exposure of urban and suburban preschool children with organic and conventional diets. Environmental Health Perspectives, 111(3): pp. 377–382. doi: 10.1289/ehp.5754

Dembinski, A., Warzecha, Z., Konturek S.J. et al. (2004): Extract of grapefruit-seed reduces acute pancreatitis induced by ischemia/reperfusion in rats: possible implication of tissue antioxidants. J Physiol Pharmacol, 55(4): pp. 811–821.

Döll, M. (2008): Die Kraft der Antioxidantien: Gesund und jung bleiben. München: Wilhelm Goldmann Verlag.

Duke, J.A. (2010): Heilende Nahrungsmittel. Wie Sie Erkrankungen mit Gemüse, Kräutern und Samen wegessen. München: Arkana.

Dumić, J., Dabelić, S. & Flögel, M. (2002): Curcumin – A Potent Inhibitor of Galectin-3 Expression. Food Technol Biotechnol, 40(4): pp. 281–287.

Dunn, S.E., Hardman, R.A., Kari, F.W. & Barrett, J.C. (1997): Insulin-like growth factor 1 (IGF-1) alters drug sensitivity of HBL100 human breast cancer cells by inhibition of apoptosis induced by diverse anticancer drugs. Cancer Res, 57(13): pp. 2687–2693.

Edwards-Jones, V., Buck, R. et al. (2004): The effect of essential oils on methicillin-resistant Staphylococcus aureus using a dressing model. Burns. 30(8): pp. 772–777.

Elmadfa, I., Aign, W., Muskat, E. & Fritzsche, D. (2015): Die große GU Nährwert-Kalorien-Tabelle. München: Gräfe und Unzer Verlag.

Folkers, K. & Simonsen, R. (1995): Two successful double-blind trials with coenzyme Q10 (vitamin Q10) on muscular dystrophies and neurogenic atrophies. Biochim Biophys Acta, 1271(1): pp. 281–286.

Frohn, B. (2013): Die Ölzieh-Kur. Einfach und wirksam entgiften. 2. Aufl., Murnau am Staffelsee: Mankau Verlag GmbH.

Fujiki, H., Suganuma, M., Okabe, S. et al. (1998): Cancer inhibition by green tea. Mutat Res, 402(1–2): pp. 307–310.

Geleijnse, J.M., Vermeer, C., Grobee, D.E. et al. (2004): Dietary intake of menaquinone is associated with a reduced risk of coronary heart disease: the Rotterdam Study. J Nutr, 134(11): pp. 3100–3105.

GFV Gesellschaft für Vitalpilzkunde e.V. (Hrsg.) (2009): Vitalpilze – Naturheilkraft mit Tradition – neu entdeckt. Gersthofen: GfV Gesellschaft für Vitalpilzkunde e.V.

Ghaffari, A.R., Noshad, H., Ostadi, A. et al. (2011): The effects of milk thistle on hepatic fibrosis due to methotrexate in rat. Hepat Mon, 11(6): pp. 464–468.

Gil, M.I., Tomás-Barberán, F.A., Hess-Pierce, B. et al. (2000): Antioxidant activity of pomegranate juice and its relationship with phenolic composition and processing. J Agric Food Chem, 48(10): pp. 4581–4589.

Gleissman, H. Johnsen, J.I. & Kogner, P. (2010): Omega-3 fatty acids in cancer, the protectors of good and the killers of evil?, Exp Cell Res, 316(8): pp. 1365–1373. doi: 10.1016/j.yexcr.2010.02.039

Goodwin, P. J., Ennis, M., Pritchard, K.I. et al. (2008): Frequency of vitamin D (Vit D) deficiency at breast cancer (BC) diagnosis and association with risk of distant recurrence and death in a prospective cohort study of T1-3, N0-1, M0 B. Journal of Clinical Oncology, 2008 ASCO Annual Meeting Proceedings (Post-Meeting Edition), Vol 26, No 15S(May 20 Supplement):511.

Grabhorn, S. (2007): Granatapfel – Frucht der Götter: Heilwirkung, Anwendungen, Tipps und Rezepte. Oy-Mittelberg: Joy Verlag GmbH.

Griffin, G.E. (2014): Eine Welt ohne Krebs: Die Geschichte des Vitamin B17 und seiner Unterdrückung. 11. Aufl., Rottenburg: Kopp Verlag.

Grothey, A., Voigt, W., Schöber, C. et al. (1999): The role of insulin-like growth factor I and its receptor in cell growth, transformation, apoptosis, and chemoresistance in solid tumors. J Cancer Res Clin Oncol, 125(3–4): pp. 166–173.

Häge, W. (2006): Biologische Krebsabwehr – Krebsprophylaxe und Krebsbehandlung durch neue Zellsymbiose-Therapien. Nienburg: Radionik Verlag.

Hauschka, P.V., Lian, J.B., Cole, D.E. & Gundberg, C.M. (1989): Osteocalcin and matrix Gla protein: vitamin K-dependent proteins in bone. Physiol Rev., 69(3): pp. 990–1047.

Heggers, J.P., Cottingham, J., Gusman, J. et al. (2002): The effectiveness of processed grapefruit-seed extract as an antibacterial agent: II. Mechanism of action and in vitro toxicity. J Altern Complement Med, 8(3): pp. 333–340.

Helène, B. (Hrsg.) (2012): Vitamin B17 – Die Revolution in der Krebsmedizin: Ein Ratgeber aus der ärztlichen Praxis nach der Dr. Puttich Krebstherapie. Books on Demand.

Herr, I. (2013): Kreuzblütler in der Krebstherapie; Aktuelle Gesundheits-Nachrichten. Heft 8/2013, pp. 52–56, Berlin: Europäische Akademie für Naturheilverfahren und Umweltmedizin (EANU).

Holick, M.F. & Jenkins, M. (2005): Schützendes Sonnenlicht: Die heilsamen Kräfte der Sonne. Stuttgart: Karl F. Haug Verlag.

Homes, G.D. (2009): Vorbeugung und Behandlung von Krebs mit Vitamin B17. www.bermibs.de/fileadmin/pdf/krebs-natuerlich_vorsorgen_und_heilen/amygdalin-vitamin_b17/vorbeugung_und_behandlung_von_krebs_mit_vitamin_b17.pdf, (last accessed September 2017).

http://blog.endokrinologie.net/fallstricke-behandlung-vitamin-d-mangel-694, (last accessed September 2017).

http://globocan.iarc.fr/Pages/fact_sheets_cancer.aspx, (last accessed September 2017).

http://nebenwirkungen.biz/2014/10/13/wie-kann-man-arginin-nebenwirkungen-vermeiden, (last accessed September 2017).

Hübner, J. & Spahn, G. (2009): Sekundäre Pflanzenstoffe. Der Onkologe, 15(11): pp. 1144–1150. doi: 10.1007/s00761-009-1729-6

Ireland, C. (2006): Hormones in milk can be dangerous. Harvard University Archives 2006 Dez 7, http://news.harvard.edu/gazette/story/2006/12/hormones-in-milk-can-be-dangerous/, (last accessed September 2017).

Irmey, G. & Jordan, A.-L. (2005): 110 wirksame Behandlungsmöglichkeiten bei Krebs. 2. Aufl., Stuttgart: Karl F. Haug Verlag.

Islami, F., Boffetta, P. & Ren, J. (2009): High-temperature beverages and Foods and Esophageal Cancer Risk -- A Systematic Review. International Journal of Cancer, 125(3), pp. 491–524. doi: 10.1002/ijc.24445

Jee, S.-H., Shen, S.-C., Tseng, C.-R. et al. (1998): Curcumin Induces a p53-Dependent Apoptosis in Human Basal Cell Carcinoma Cells. Journal of Investigative Dermatology, 111(4), pp. 656–661. doi: 10.1046/j.1523-1747.1998.00352.x

Jehle, S., Hulter, H.N. & Krapf, R. (2013): Effect of potassium citrate on bone density, microarchitecture, and fracture risk in healthy older adults without Osteoporosis: a randomized controlled trial. J Clin Endocrinol Metab, 98(1): pp. 207–217. doi: 10.1210/jc.2012–3099

Jehle, S., Zanetti, A., Muser, J. et al. (2006): Partial neutralization of the acidogenic western diet with potassium citrate increases bone mass in postmenopausal women with osteopenia. J Am Soc Nephrol, 17(11): pp. 3213–3222. doi: 10.1681/ASN.2006030233

Jensen, B. (2002): Der Fruchtsaft-Doktor: Gesundheit und ein langes Leben mit der Kraft der Vitamine. München: Mosaik/Wilhelm Goldmann Verlag.

Jugdaohsingh, R., Tucker, K.L., Qiao, N. et al. (2004): Dietary silicon intake is positively associated with bone mineral density in men and premenopausal women of the Framingham Offspring cohort. J Bone Miner Res, 19(2): pp. 297–307.

Kanai, M., Imaizumi, A., Otsuka, Y. et al. (2012): Dose-escalation and pharmacokinetic study of nanoparticle curcumin, a potential anticancer agent with improved bioavailability, in healthy human volunteers. Cancer Chemother Pharmacol, 69(1): pp. 65–70. doi: 10.1007/s00280-011-1673-1

Kaufhold, P. (2012): PhytoMagister – Zu den Wurzeln der Kräuterheilkunst. Modernes und traditionelles Wissen der Pflanzenheilkunde für Praxis und Unterricht. Bd. 2, 5. Aufl., Norderstedt: Books on Demand GmbH.

Kern, P. (2014): Krebs bekämpfen mit Vitamin B17: Vorbeugen und Heilen mit Nitrilen aus Aprikosenkernen. 8. Aufl., Kirchzarten: VAK Verlags GmbH.

Khajehdehi, P., Zanjaninejad, B., Aflaki, E. et al. (2012): Oral supplementation of turmeric decreases proteinuria, hematuria, and systolic blood pressure in patients suffering from relapsing or refractory lupus nephritis: a randomized and placebo-controlled study. J Ren Nutr, 22(1): 50–57. doi: 10.1053/j.jrn.2011.03.002

Khayat, D. (2011): Stark gegen Krebs: Wie Sie sich mit der richtigen Ernährung schützen. München: Wilhelm Goldmann Verlag.

Kiremidjian-Schumacher, L., Roy, M., Wishe, H.I. et al. (1994): Supplementation with selenium and human immune cell functions. II. Effect on cytotoxic lymphocytes and natural killer cells. Biol Trace Elem Res, 41(1–2): pp. 115–127.

Knasmüller, S. (2014): Krebs und Ernährung: Risiken und Prävention – wissenschaftliche Grundlagen und Ernährungsempfehlungen. Stuttgart: Georg Thieme Verlag KG.

Kooncumchoo, P., Sharma, S., Porter, J. et al. (2006): Coenzyme Q10 provides neuroprotection in iron-induced apoptosis in dopaminergic neurons. J Mol Neurosci, 28(2): pp. 125–141.

Krajewska-Kułak, E., Lukaszuk, C. & Niczyporuk, W. (2001): [Effects of 33% grapefruit extract on the growth of the yeast--like fungi, dermatopytes and moulds] [Article in Polish]. Wiad Parazytol, 47(4): pp. 845–849.

Küçükgergin, C., Aydin, A.F., Özdemirler-Erata, G. et al. (2010): Effect of artichoke leaf extract on hepatic and cardiac oxidative stress in rats fed on high cholesterol diet. Biol Trace Elem Res, 135(13): pp. 264–274. doi: 10.1007/s12011-009-8484-9

Kundu, J.K. & Surh, Y.-J. (2012): Emerging avenues linking inflammation and cancer. Free Radic Biol Med, 52(9): pp. 2013–2037. doi: 10.1016/j.freeradbiomed.2012.02.035

Labrecque, L., Lamy, S., Chapus, A. et al. (2005): Combined inhibition of PDGF and VEGF receptors by ellagic acid, a dietary-derived phenolic compound. Carcinogenesis, 26(4): pp. 821–826.

Lambert, H., Frassetto, L., Moore, J.B. et al. (2015): The effect of supplementation with alkaline potassium salts on bone metabolism: a meta-analysis. Osteoporos Int, 26(4): pp. 1311–1318. doi: 10.1007/s00198-014-3006-9

Lane, D.P. (1992): p53, guardian of the genome. Nature, 358(6381), pp. 15–16. doi: 10.1038/358015a0

Lappe, J.M., Travers-Gustafson, D., Davies, K.M. et al. (2007): Vitamin D and calcium supplementation reduces cancer risk: results of a randomized trial. Am J Clin Nutr, 85(6): pp. 1586–1591.

Li, Y., Zhang, T., Korkaya, H. et al. (2010): Sulforaphane, a dietary component of broccoli/broccoli sprouts, inhibits breast cancer stem cells. Clin Cancer Res, 16(9): pp. 2580–2590. doi: 10.1158/1078-0432.CCR-09-2937

lmai, K., Matsuyama, S., Miyake, S. et al. (2000): Natural cytotoxic activity of peripheral-blood lymphocytes and cancer incidence: an 11-year follow-up study of a general population. Lancet, 356(9244): pp. 1795–1799.

Lodish, H., Baltimore, D., Berk, A. et al. (1996): Molekulare Zellbiologie. 2. Aufl., Berlin: Walter de Gruyter & Co.

Long, L., Navab, R. & Brodt, P. (1998): Regulation of the Mr 72,000 type IV collagenase by the type I insulin-like growth factor receptor. Cancer Res, 58(15): pp. 3243–3247.

Makarevic, J., Rutz, J., Juengel, E. et al. (2014): Amygdalin Blocks Bladder Cancer Cell Growth in vitro by Diminishing Cyclin A and cdk2. PLoS ONE 9(8):e105590. doi:10.1371/journal.pone.0105590

Mandal, V., Dewanjee, S., Sahu, R., Mandal, S.C. et al. (2009): Design and optimization of ultrasound assisted extraction of curcumin as an effective alternative for conventional solid liquid extraction of natural products. Nat Prod Commun, 4(1): pp. 95–100.

Martin, K.R. (2013): Silicon: The Health Benefits of a Metalloid. In: Interrelations between Essential Metal Ions and Human Diseases. Sigel, A., Sigel, H., Sigel, R.K.O. (Hrsg.), Metal Ions in Life Sciences, 13: pp. 451–473. doi: 10.1007/978-94-007-7500-8_14

Masterjohn, C. (2007): Vitamin D toxicity redefined: vitamin K and the molecular mechanism. Med Hypotheses. 68(5): pp. 1026–1034. doi: 10.1016/j.mehy.2006.09.051

Meyer, R.H.P. (2010): Chronisch gesund (Prinzipien einer Gesundheitspraxis). 5. Aufl.

Narayanan, B.A., Geoffroy, O., Willingham, M.C. et al. (1999): p53/p21 (WAF1/CIP1) expression and its possible role in G1 arrest and apoptosis in ellagic acid treated cancer cells. Cancer Lett, 136(2): pp. 215–221. doi: 10.1016/S0304-3835(98)00323-1

Nesterenko, S. (2010): Entgiften von A bis Z: Wie Sie Ihren Körper von Schwermetallen und anderen Umweltschadstoffen befreien. Rainer Bloch Verlag.

Niederer, M. (2012): Gesund von Geburt an: Natürliche Anfangsnahrung. Books on Demand.

Nimptsch, K., Rohrmann, S. & Linseisen, J. (2008): Dietary intake of vitamin K and risk of prostate cancer in the Heidelberg cohort of the European Prospective Investigation into Cancer and Nutrition (EPIC-Heidelberg). Am J Clin Nutr, 87(4): pp. 985–992.

Nimptsch, K., Rohrmann, S., Kaaks, R. & Linseisen, J. (2010): Dietary vitamin K intake in relation to cancer incidence and mortality: results from the Heidelberg cohort of the European Prospective Investigation into Cancer and Nutrition (EPIC-Heidelberg). Am J Clin Nutr, 91(5): pp. 1348–1358. doi: 10.3945/ajcn.2009.28691

Nöcker, R.-M. (2004): Das große Buch der Sprossen und Keime. Mit vielen Rezepten. 7. Auflage, München: Wilhelm Heyne Verlag GmbH.

Oates, L., Cohen, M., Braun, L. et al. (2014): Reduction in urinary organophosphate pesticide metabolites in adults after a week-long organic diet. Environ Res, 132: pp. 105–111. doi: 10.1016/j.envres.2014.03.021

Ooi, V.E.C. & Liu, F. (2000): Immunomodulation and anti-cancer activity of polysaccharide-protein complexes. Curr Med Chem, 7(7): pp. 715–29.

Ovadje, P., Chatterjee, S., Griffin, C. et al. (2011): Selective induction of apoptosis through activation of caspase-8 in human leukemia cells (Jurkat) by dandelion root extract. J Ethnopharmacol, 133(1): pp. 86–91. doi: 10.1016/j.jep.2010.09.005

Ovadje, P., Chochkeh, M., Akbari-Asl, P. et al. (2012): Selective induction of apoptosis and autophagy through treatment with dandelion root extract in human pancreatic cancer cells. Pancreas, 41(7): pp. 1039–1047. doi: 10.1097/MPA.0b013e31824b22a2

Paller, C.J., Ye, X., Wozniak, P.J. et al. (2013): A randomized phase II study of pomegranate extract for men with rising PSA following initial therapy for localized prostate cancer. Prostate Cancer Prostatic Dis, 16(1): pp. 50–55. doi: 10.1038/pcan.2012.20

Pantuck, A.J., Leppert, J.T., Zomorodian, N. et al. (2006): Phase II study of pomegranate juice for men with rising prostate-specific antigen following surgery or radiation for prostate cancer. Clin Cancer Res, 12(13): pp. 4018–4026. doi: 10.1158/1078–0432.CCR-05–2290

Parkin, D.M., Bray, F., Ferlay, J. & Pisani, P. (2005): Global cancer statistics, 2002. CA Cancer J Clin. 55(2): pp. 74–108.

Pientka, A. (2007): Prognostische Bedeutung klinisch-pathologischer Faktoren beim adenoidzystischen Karzinom des Kopf-Hals-Bereiches. Eine retrospektive Untersuchung am Patientengut der Klinik für Hals-, Nasen- und Ohrenheilkunde der Philipps-Universität Marburg. Dissertation. Philipps-Universität Marburg.

Potter, G.A. & Burke, M.D. (2006): Salvestrols – Natural Products with Tumour Selective Activity. Journal of Orthomolecular Medicine, 21(1): pp. 34–36.

Potter, G.A., Patterson, L.H., Wanogho, E. et al. (2002): The cancer preventative agent resveratrol is converted to the anticancer agent piceatannol by the cytochrome P450 enzyme CYP1B1. Br J Cancer, 86(5): pp. 774–778.

Puspitasari, I.M., Abdulah, R., Yamazaki, C. et al. (2014): Updates on clinical studies of selenium supplementation in radiotherapy. Radiation Oncology, 9:125. doi: 10.1186/1748–717X-9–125

Rausch, V., Liu, L., Kallifatidis, G. et al. (2010): Synergistic activity of sorafenib and sulforaphane abolishes pancreatic cancer stem cell characteristics. Cancer Res, 70(12): pp. 5004–5013. doi: 10.1158/0008–5472.CAN-10–0066

Raven, P.H., Ray, F.E. & Eichhorn, S.E. (2006): Primäre und sekundäre Pflanzenstoffe. In: Biologie der Pflanzen. 4. Aufl., Berlin: Walter de Gruyter GmbH und Co. KG.

Reagor, L., Gusman, J., McCoy, L. et al. (2002): The effectiveness of processed grapefruit-seed extract as an antibacterial agent: I. An in vitro agar assay. J Altern Complement Med, 8(3): pp. 325–332.

Reddy, M.K., Gupta, S.K., Jacob, M.R. et al. (2007): Antioxidant, antimalarial and antimicrobial activities of tannin-rich fractions, ellagitannins and phenolic acids from Punica granatum L. Planta Med. 73(5): pp. 461–467.

Reuter, U. & Oettmeier, R. (2005): Biologische Krebsbehandlung heute. Sag' ja zum Leben. 2. Aufl., Greiz: Akademie und Fachverlag im LEBEN OHG.

Ribeiro, C.A.O., Vollaire, Y., Sanchez-Chardi, A. & Roche, H. (2005): Bioaccumulation and the effects of organochlorine pesticides, PAH and heavy metals in the Eel (Anguilla anguilla) at the Camargue Nature Reserve, France. Aquat Toxicol, 74(1): pp. 53–69. doi: 10.1016/j.aquatox.2005.04.008

Riedl, R. & Lütgendorff-Gyllenstorm, H. (2011): Zu heißes Essen und Trinken – die unbeachtete Gefahr. Deutsche Lebensmittel-Rundschau, 107(2): pp. 71–83B.

Sánchez, Á.C. & Barrachina, A.A.C.: Der Granatapfel aus Spanien. Antioxidative Eigenschaften des Punicalagins im Saft und Extrakt des Granatapfels, in der funktionalen Ernährung der Zukunft.

Santel, T., Pflug, G., Hemdan, N.Y.A. et al. (2008): Curcumin Inhibits Glyoxalase 1: a possible link to its anti-inflammatory and anti-tumor activity. PLoS One, 3(10): e3508. doi: 10.1371/journal.pone.0003508

Schaefer, B.A., Hoon, L.T., Burke, M.D. & Potter, G.A. (2007): Nutrition and Cancer: Salvestrol Case Studies. Journal of Orthomolecular Medicine, 22(4): pp. 177–182.

Schaefer, B.A., Potter, G.A., Wood, R. et al. (2012): Cancer and Related Case Studies Involving Salvestrol and CYP1B1. Journal of Orthomolecular Medicine, Vol. 27(3): pp. 131–138.

Schleicher, P. & Saleh, M. (2007): Natürlich heilen mit Schwarzkümmelöl. Die besten Anwendungen, um körpereigene Abwehrkräfte zu aktivieren. 6. Aufl., München: Südwest Verlag.

Schmelzer, C., Lindner, I., Rimbach, G. et al. (2008): Functions of coenzyme Q10 in inflammation and gene expression. BioFactors, 32(1–4): pp. 179–183.

Schurgers, L.J., Knapen, M.H.J. & Vermeer, C. (2007): Vitamin K2 improves bone strength in postmenopausal women. International Congress Series, Vol. 1297, pp. 179–187. doi: 10.1016/j.ics.2006.08.006

Schwarz, G. (2011): Gesund mit Sauerkraut und Kohl: Immunstärkend – Entgiftend – Darmregulierend. München: F.A. Herbig Verlagsbuchhandlung GmbH.

Servan-Schreiber, D. (2012): Das Antikrebs-Buch: Was uns schützt: Vorbeugen und Nachsorgen mit natürlichen Mitteln. 6. Aufl., München: Wilhelm Goldmann Verlag.

Seyfried, T.N. & Shelton, L.M. (2010): Cancer as a metabolic disease. Nutr Metab, 7:7. doi: 10.1186/1743-7075-7-7

Shargorodsky, M., Debby, O., Matas, Z. & Zimlichman, R. (2010): Effect of long-term treatment with antioxidants (vitamin C, vitamin E, coenzyme Q10 and selenium) on arterial compliance, humoral factors and inflammatory markers in patients with multiple cardiovascular risk factors. Nutrition & Metabolism, 7:55. doi: 10.1186/1743-7075-7-55

Shoba, G., Joy, D., Joseph, T. et al. (1998): Influence of piperine on the pharmacokinetics of curcumin in animals and human volunteers. Planta Med, 64(4): pp. 353–356.

Sigstedt, S.C., Hooten, C.J., Callewaert, M.C. et al. (2008): Evaluation of aqueous extracts of Taraxacum officinale on growth and invasion of breast and prostate cancer cells. Int J Oncol, 32(5): pp. 1085–1090. doi: 10.3892/ijo.32.5.1085

Simonsohn, B. (2008): Heilkraft aus den Tropen: Die süße Medizin exotischer Früchte. München: Integral Verlag.

Skinner, H.G. & Schwartz, G.G. (2008): Serum calcium and incident and fatal prostate cancer in the National Health and Nutrition Examination Survey. Cancer Epidemiol Biomarkers Prev, 17(9): pp. 2302–2305. doi: 10.1158/1055–9965.EPI-08-0365

Song, Z. & Xu, X. (2014): Advanced research on anti-tumor effects of amygdalin. J Cancer Res Ther, 10(5): pp. 3–7. doi: 10.4103/0973–1482.139743

Tomé, D. & Bos, C. (2007): Lysine requirement through the human life cycle. J Nutr, 137(6 Suppl 2): pp. 1642S–1645S.

Treutwein, N. (2001): Übersäuerung – Krank ohne Grund. München: Südwest Verlag.

Vermeer, C., Jie, K.-S.G. & Knapen, M.H.J. (1995): Role of vitamin K in bone metabolism. Annu Rev Nutr, 15: pp. 1–22.

Wagner, H. (1995): Krebs mit Schwarzkümmelöl vorgebeugt: Uraltes Naturmittel von der High-Tech-Medizin neu entdeckt. 14. 9. 1995, welt.de, www.welt.de/print-welt/article662113/Krebs-mit-Schwarzkuemmeloel-vorgebeugt.html, (last accessed September 2017).

Watzl, B. & Leitzmann, C. (2005): Bioaktive Substanzen in Lebensmitteln. 3. Aufl., Stuttgart: Hippokrates Verlag.

Weuffen, W. & Decker, H. (2004): Thiocyanat – ein bioaktives Ion mit orthomolekularem Charakter. Sarow: I.S.M.H. Verlag.

www.adler-muehle.de/info/Weizenkorn.html, (last accessed September 2017).

www.aminosaeuren.biz/l-lysin, (last accessed September 2017).

www.cancertutor.com/dandelionroot, (last accessed September 2017).

www.chemie.de/lexikon/Kollagen.html, (last accessed September 2017).

www.dge.de/wissenschaft/weitere-publikationen/ fachinformationen/rauchen-und-koerpergewicht, (last accessed September 2017).

www.drjacobsinstitut.de/?Prostatakarzinom/ Knochenmetastasen, (last accessed September 2017).

www.faux.at/Vitamin%20D%20Quellen, (last accessed September 2017).

www.fh-erfurt.de/lgf/fileadmin/GB/Dokumente/ Forschung/Bioaktive_Substanzen_im_Gemuese.pdf, (last accessed September 2017).

www.gesundheit.com/gc_detail_7_gc01070218.html, (last accessed September 2017).

www.gesundheit.de/ernaehrung/gesund-essen/ ernaehrungswissen/sekundaere-pflanzenstoffe-was-sind-das-eigentlich-fuer-stoffe, (last accessed September 2017).

www.gesundheit.gv.at/Portal.Node/ghp/public/content/ labor/referenzwerte/Vitamin_D_125_Dihydroxy-vitamin-D_VD125_HK.html, (last accessed September 2017).

www.gruenertee.de/inhaltsstoffe/polyphenole-im-gruenen-tee, (last accessed September 2017).

www.gruenertee.de/wirkung/krebs, (last accessed September 2017).

www.klinikum.uni-heidelberg.de/fuer-Patienten.111688.0.html, (last accessed September 2017).

www.klinikum.uni-heidelberg.de/Wie-wirkt-Sulforaphan.138791.0.html, (last accessed September 2017).

www.lebensmittellexikon.de/g0000620.php, (last accessed September 2017).

www.naturheilkunde-lexikon.eu/lexikon-naturheilkunde/ lexikon-s/salvestrole, (last accessed March 2016).

www.naturheilpraxis-hollmann.de/Immunstatus_Grosser. htm, (last accessed September 2017).

www.nikotinpraevention.de/was_wir_wollen/ wissenschaftskritik.html, (last accessed September 2017).

www.nu3.at/blog/kokoswasser-inhaltsstoffe, (last accessed September 2017).

www.orthoknowledge.eu/fachinformation-uber-die-aminosauren-lysin-und-prolin-sowie-uber-entkoffeinierten-gruntee-extrakt, (last accessed September 2017).

www.orthoknowledge.eu/vitamin-k-vielseitiger-als-bisher-gedacht, (last accessed September 2017).

www.osteoporosezentrum.de/vitamin-d-metabolite-knochenaufbaustimulierende-medikamente-einnahmevorschriften-von-vitamin-d-metabolite/, (last accessed September 2017).

www.paracelsus-magazin.de/alle-ausgaben/56-heft-062011/766-grapefruitkernextrakt.html, (last accessed September 2017).

www.scientistlive.com/content/20610, (last accessed September 2017).

www.sein.de/guolin-qigong-wirksame-hilfe-bei-krebs, (last accessed September 2017).

www.swiss-paediatrics.org/sites/default/files/paediatrica/ vol23/n4/pdf/11.pdf, (last accessed September 2017).

www.vitamind.net/vitamin-k, (last accessed September 2017).

www.webmed.ch/docs/selen/Selen_Teil_I.htm, (last accessed September 2017).

www.zentrum-der-gesundheit.de/enzymtherapie.html, (last accessed September 2017).

www.zentrum-der-gesundheit.de/grapefruitkernextrakt. html, (last accessed September 2017).

www.zuckerverbaende.de/zuckermarkt/zahlen-und-fakten/weltzuckermarkt/erzeugung-verbrauch.html, (last accessed September 2017).

www4ger.dr-rath-foundation.org/NATUERLICHE_
GESUNDHEIT/zellular_medizin/krebs.html,
(last accessed September 2017).

Yallapu, M.M., Maher, D.M., Sundram, V. et al. (2010):
Curcumin induces chemo/radio-sensitization in
ovarian cancer cells and curcumin nanoparticles
inhibit ovarian cancer cell growth. J Ovarian Res, 3:11.
doi: 10.1186/1757-2215-3-11

Yumen, H. (2010): Untersuchungen über Polyphenole
in weißen und grünen Tees. Dissertation. Technische
Universität Carolo-Wilhelmina, Braunschweig.

Zagermann-Muncke, P. (2005): Grapefruit und
Arzneimittel. www.pharmazeutische-zeitung.de/index.
php?id=pharm1_31_2005, (last accessed September
2017).

The environment and the immune system

Brodin, P., Jojic, V., Gao, T. et al. (2015): Variation in the
Hu-man Immune System Is Largely Driven by Non-
Heritable Influences. Cell. Vol. 160(Issues 1-2): pp. 37-47.
doi: http://dx.doi.org/10.1016/j.cell.2014.12.020

The mind influences our immune system

Ehlert, U. (2016): Verhaltensmedizin. 2. Aufl., Berlin:
Springer.

Futterman, A.D., Kemeny, M.E., Shapiro, D. & Fahey, J.L. (1994): Immunological and physiological changes associated with induced positive and negative mood. Psychosom Med, 56(6): pp. 499–511.

Hermes, G.L., Delgado, B., Tretiakova, M. et al. (2009): Social isolation dysregulates endocrine and behavioral stress while increasing malignant burden of spontaneous mammary tumors. Proc Natl Acad Sci U S A, 106(52): pp. 22393–22398. doi: 10.1073/pnas.0910753106

Schubert, C. (2011): Von der Psyche zum Immunsystem und zurück. 25. 1. 2011, SpringerMedizin.at, www.springermedizin.at/artikel/20489-von-der-psyche-zum-immunsystem-und-zurueck, (last accessed September 2017).

Visintainer, M.A., Volpicelli, J.R. & Seligman, M.E. (1982): Tumor rejection in rats after inescapable or escapable shock. Science. 216(4544): pp. 437–439.

Physical activity and the immune system

Beuth, J. (2011): Gesund bleiben nach Krebs: Was Sie jetzt stärkt und schützt – Was hilft und einen Rückfall abwehrt. München: Wilhelm Goldmann Verlag.

Coy, J.F., Baumann, F.T., Spitz, J. & Cavelius, A. (2011): Die 8 Anti-Krebs-Regeln: Gesund im Einklang mit unseren steinzeitlichen Genen. München: Gräfe und Unzer Verlag GmbH.

Haber, P. (2009): Leitfaden zur medizinischen Trainingsberatung. Rehabilitation bis Leistungssport. 3. Aufl., Wien: Springer-Verlag.

Sephton, S. & Spiegel, D. (2003): Circadian disruption in cancer: a neuroendocrine-immune pathway from stress to disease? Brain, Behavior, and Immunity, Vol. 17(5), pp. 321–328.

Straif, K., Baan, R., Grosse, Y. et al. (2007): Carcinogenicity of shift-work, painting, and fire-fighting. The Lancet Oncology, Vol. 8(12), pp. 1065–1066. doi: 10.1016/S1470-2045(07)70373-X

www.krankheiten.de/laborwerte/leukozyten.php, (last accessed September 2017).

www.leukozyten-info.de/leukozyten-erhoehen.html, (last accessed September 2017).

www.runnersnews.de/wissenswertes/frauen.htm, (last accessed March 2016).

How I dealt with the side effects

Clegg, D.O., Reda, D.J., Harris, C.L. et al. (2006): Glucosamine, chondroitin sulfate, and the two in combination for painful knee osteoarthritis. N Engl J Med, 354(8): pp. 795–808.

Cronin, J. R. (1999): Methylsulfonylmethane – Nutraceutical of the next century? Alternative and Complementary Therapies, 5(6): pp. 386–389. doi: 10.1089/act.1999.5.386

Debbi, E.M., Agar, G., Fichman, G. et al. (2011): Efficacy of methylsulfonylmethane supplementation on osteoarthritis of the knee: a randomized controlled study. BMC Complement Altern Med, 11:50. doi: 10.1186/1472-6882-11-50

Deutsch, L. (2007): Evaluation of the effect of Neptune Krill Oil on chronic inflammation and arthritic symptoms. J Am Coll Nutr, 26(1): pp. 39–48.

Dhivya, H. (2012): Glutathione – a master antioxidant and an immune system modulator. Journal of Biological and Information Sciences; Vol.1, Iss. 3: pp. 28–30.

Döll, M. (2015): Arthrose: Endlich schmerzfrei durch Naturheilmittel. München: Wilhelm Goldmann Verlag.

Gradelet, S., Le Bon, A.-M., Bergès, R. et al. (1998): Dietary carotenoids inhibit aflatoxin B1-induced liver preneoplastic foci and DNA damage in the rat: role of the modulation of aflatoxin B1 metabolism. Carcinogenesis, 19(3): pp. 403–411.

Guerin, M., Huntley, M.E. & Olaizola, M. (2003): Haematococcus astaxanthin: applications for human health and nutrition. Trends Biotechnol, 21(5): pp. 210–216.

http://chirurgie.uniklinikumgraz.at/thorax_und_hyperbare_chirurgie/Abteilung/Druckkammer/Seiten/default.aspx, (last accessed September 2017).

http://natur-wissen.com/wp-content/uploads/2014/04/Gelenkschmerzen-Was-Sie-unbedingt-wissen-sollten.pdf, (last accessed September 2017).

www.gtuem.org/77/druckkammern/hbo-therapie, (last accessed September 2017).

www.klinikum-graz.at/cms/dokumente/10309483_9124185/d69f5c23/PM_Nach%20Genickbruch%20kann%20Patientin%20wieder%20gehen.pdf, (last accessed September 2017).

Jacob, S.W., Lawrence, R.M.& Zucker, M. (1999): The Miracle of MSM: The Natural Solution for Pain. New York: Berkley Books.

Kim, L.S., Axelrod, L.J., Howard, P. et al. (2006): Efficacy of methylsulfonylmethane (MSM) in osteoarthritis pain of the knee: a pilot clinical trial. Osteoarthritis Cartilage, 14(3): pp. 286–294. doi: 10.1016/j.joca.2005.10.003

Kindwall, E.P. (1995): Hyperbaric Medicine Practice. Flagstaff: Best Publishing.

Kroboth, P.D., Amico, J.A., Stone, R.A. et al. (2003): Influence of DHEA administration on 24-hour cortisol concentrations. J Clin Psychopharmacol, 23(1): pp. 96–99.

Kurashige, M., Okimasu, E., Inoue, M. & Utsumi, K. (1990): Inhibition of oxidative injury of biological membranes by astaxanthin. Physiol Chem Phys Med NMR, 22(1): pp. 27–38.

Parcell, S. (2002): Sulfur in human nutrition and applications in medicine. Altern Med Rev, 7(1): pp. 22–44.

Park, J.S., Chyun, J.H., Kim, Y.K. et al. (2010): Astaxanthin decreased oxidative stress and inflammation and enhanced immune response in humans. Nutrition & Metabolism, 7:18. doi: 10.1186/1743-7075-7-18

Pschyrembel, W. (2004): Psychrembel. Klinisches Wörterbuch. 260. Aufl., Berlin: Walter de Gruyter.

Schomakers, S. (2008): Hirndrucksenkende Maßnahmen. Oktober 2008, Universitätsklinikum Münster, http:// klinikum.uni-muenster.de/fileadmin/ukminternet/ daten/zentralauftritt/ukm-mitarbeiter/schulen_ weiterbildung/anin/arbeiten/intensivpflege_anaesthesie/ Hirndrucksenkende_Massnahmen_2009.pdf,   (last accessed September 2017).

Striebel, H.W. (2008): Operative Intensivmedizin: Sicherheit in der klinischen Praxis. Stuttgart: Schattauer GmbH.

Tripathi, D.N. & Jena, G.B. (2010): Astaxanthin intervention ameliorates cyclophosphamide-induced oxidative stress, DNA damage and early hepatocarcinogenesis in rat: Role of Nrf2, p53, p38 and phase-II enzymes. Mutat Res, 696(1): pp. 69–80. doi: 10.1016/j.mrgentox.2009.12.014

Usha, P.R. & Naidu, M.U.R. (2004): Randomised, Double-Blind, Parallel, Placebo-Controlled Study of Oral Glucosamine, Methylsulfonylmethane and their Combination in Osteoarthritis. Clin Drug Invest, 24(6): pp. 353–363.

Vangsness, C.T., Spiker, W. & Erickson, J. (2009): Arthroscopy, 25(1): pp. 86–94. doi: 10.1016/j.arthro.2008.07.020

www.hirntumorhilfe.at/hirntumor/hirntumortherapie/strahlentherapie/strahlennekrose, (last accessed September 2017).

www.krebsinformationsdienst.de/behandlung/strahlentherapie-biologie.php, (last accessed September 2017).

www.medizinfo.de/arzneimittel/resorption/schranken.shtml, (last accessed September 2017).

www.orthoknowledge.eu/astaxanthin-ein-sehr-wirkungsvolles-und-vielseitiges-carotinoid, (last accessed September 2017).

www.rheuma-liga.de/fileadmin/user_upload/Dokumente/Hilfe_bei_Rheuma/Therapie/Medikamententherapie/kortison/medikamentenfuehrer_3.pdf, (last accessed September 2017).

Made in the USA
Middletown, DE
12 September 2018